MEG HICKLING'S
grown-up
sex

SEXUAL WHOLENESS
FOR THE BETTER PART
OF YOUR LIFE

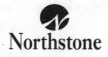

Northstone

Editor: Mike Schwartzentruber
Cover and interior design: Verena Velten and Margaret Kyle
Prepress Production: Chaunda Daigneault
Proofreader: Dianne Greenslade
Cover art: © iStock with adaptation
Anatomical drawings pp. 33, 46: Susan Neill, © 2008 Wood Lake Publishing Inc.

Permissions

"Paean" by Jill Dawson © Jill Dawson 1992. Reproduced from *The Virago Book of Wicked Verse* edited by Jill Dawson used by kind permission of Virago, an imprint of Little, Brown Book Group.

"The Lover" by Solveig Von Schoultz, translated by Anne Born. Translation copyright Anne Born. Used by permission.

Northstone is an imprint of Wood Lake Publishing, Inc. Wood Lake Publishing acknowledges the financial support of the Government of Canada, through the Book Publishing Industry Development Program (BPIDP) for its publishing activities. Wood Lake Publishing also acknowledges the financial support of the Province of British Columbia through the Book Publishing Tax Credit.

At Wood Lake Publishing, we practise what we publish, being guided by a concern for fairness, justice, and equal opportunity in all of our relationships with employees and customers. Wood Lake Publishing is an employee-owned company, committed to caring for the environment and all creation. Wood Lake Publishing recycles, reuses, and encourages readers to do the same. Resources are printed on 100% post-consumer recycled paper and more environmentally friendly groundwood papers (newsprint), whenever possible. A percentage of all profit is donated to charitable organizations.

Library and Archives Canada Cataloguing in Publication
Hickling, Meg, 1941-
    Meg Hickling's grown-up sex: sexual wholeness for the better part of
your life / [Meg Hickling].
Includes bibliographical references.
ISBN 978-1-55145-567-9
    1. Sex. 2. Sex customs. 3. Hygiene, Sexual. 4. Middle-aged
persons--Sexual behavior. I. Title.
HQ21.H53 2008   306.7   C2008-904009-0

Published by Northstone
An imprint of Wood Lake Publishing Inc.
9590 Jim Bailey Road, Kelowna, BC, Canada, V4V 1R2
www.woodlakebooks.com
250.766.2778

Printing 10 9 8 7 6 5 4 3 2 1
Printed in Canada by Friesens

DEDICATION

To my husband of 45 years, Tony Hickling.

And to my editor of 11 years,
Michael Schwartzentruber,
whose editing cannot be matched.

TABLE OF CONTENTS

INTRODUCTION

The Search for Sexual Maturity

The first sex manual was written in 2700 BCE by the Taoist Yellow Emperor and thousands of such texts have been published since then. This is not a sex manual.

This is a book that I hope will begin to address a searching for wholeness around sexuality that I have heard expressed by many people during more than 30 years of teaching sexual health.

My students have ranged in age from three to 99. They have come from all levels of education, and from a great many professions, cultures, and faith backgrounds. As a teacher and as an author, I have been privileged to hear their personal stories – stories that reflect joy and that celebrate positive sexual experiences; as well as stories that tell of horror, shame, and pain around sexuality. I hope that you will find inspiration, enlightenment, courage, and goodwill in the stories that I share here.

I think it is important, too, to say that I am not a doctor or a registered therapist. I am a nurse. Please seek medical or emotional care from a professional, if you experience a need for assistance as you read the book.

SEXUAL MATURITY

It is not always easy to articulate or define sexual maturity in our Western societies. I believe that we need to recognize how pervasive sexual issues are in our cultures, and to learn how a sexually mature person responds to these issues. I would ask you to work on your own definition of sexual maturity as you read through the chapters that follow.

HEALING

This book is meant to be subversive and it will not thrill everyone. There is humour here, to be sure, and there are ideas for reflection. But there is also chiding of institutions.

Most of all, I hope that there is healing where it is needed. I do not want to judge individuals. Rather, I seek to offer the kind of compassion and hope that will overcome shame and guilt. I want to offer illumination, too, to those who feel uneducated. So often, people in my audiences have said, "I feel so embarrassed. I didn't know half of what you taught us today." Typically, I respond, "How were you supposed to learn when no one ever talked to you at home, at school, in church or temple, or in the doctor's office, or printed this information in a newspaper?" Many people who were raised in homes and communities that repressed sexuality never give themselves permission to think about or to research information on these topics.

I believe we all want a world where everyone can live gracefully, with dignity, and with equality and goodwill. Over the course of my career as a sexual health educator, I have found that there is a great need for healing and an even greater need to prevent sexual trauma in the first place so that healing is not needed. Sexual health education is one way to prevent sexual trauma and sometimes it is a path to healing as well.

THE HEALING POWER OF STORIES

I have learned over the years that stories hold immense power to heal, which is one reason why I enjoy telling them so much. Although the following incident involves the healing of a child, I share it here because I find that it speaks powerfully to adults, perhaps because it addresses the wounded child inside so many of us.

I was teaching in a Grade 7 classroom. At the back of room there was a desk that was much larger than all the others. One of the students, a boy, had had a growth spurt far ahead of the other 12- and 13-year-olds, so this was his desk. The teacher sat nearby.

In my teaching sessions with grade-school children, I always tell them a story about how a baby grows in the uterus, inside the "water bag." As I began to open my three-dimensional picture of a uterus and of an about-to-be-born baby, I talked about the contractions of labour: "The uterus begins to contract and relax, giving the baby great big hugs, until after several hours of hugs, the water bag breaks and the baby comes out of the vagina, like a waterslide."

All of the children were smiling and hugging themselves, except for the big boy at the back of the room. He put his head down on his arms and his shoulders were shaking with silent sobs. I kept on talking about post-birth care, because I didn't want to have the others notice his distress. I saw the teacher kneel beside the boy and whisper to him. He seemed to reply, and, for a minute or so, she gently rubbed his back. Eventually, he raised his head, wiped away his tears, smiled at me, and continued listening. He even asked a question when we talked about puberty changes later in the class.

After the class had been dismissed for lunch, I asked the teacher what had happened.

She said, "Oh, that's Trevor. His mother died a few hours after he was born. I think it was one of those rare blood clots." She went on: "His father has done a great job raising him; he's a very bright boy, shy and quiet, but very nice."

"But why was he crying?" I asked.

"I asked him if he was okay and he said, 'Yes, I'm all right. It's just that I never knew how much my mom loved me before she died.'"

Of course, both the teacher and I were in tears by this time!

The next year, when I was back at that school, I asked the teacher about Trevor. She said, "I haven't seen him since he went to high school, but I know he's fine. His dad came to see me at the end of the school year to thank me for 'whatever you did to help Trevor.'"

It seems that Trevor had become much less shy, had joined a baseball team for the first time, had begun to excel at music and was participating in recitals, and was so much more "comfortable in his own skin."

The teacher said she told him it wasn't anything she had done: "It was Meg."

I, in turn, told the teacher that it wasn't me. It was the story about the "hugs" he received when he was in his mother's uterus.

As I said, stories can heal very deep wounds. Sometimes, the stories we need to hear so that healing can happen come from our own lives or from the lives of those closest to us.

Many abuse survivors have a heightened fear of touch that may seem nonsensical or irrational to others.

A few years ago, during a coffee break in a presentation to a group of parents, I was alone in the room and a woman returned to me from the coffee area. She began to tell me a story that she had never told anyone before. She said that one day, when she was six years old and on her way home from school, a man approached her. He began talking to her, telling her how beautiful her long, dark hair was. As he stroked the back of her head, he exposed his penis. Fortunately, she broke free and ran with all her strength until she was home.

As was the case with many youngsters of her generation, sexuality was never spoken about in her Roman Catholic home or at her school. And so, as a young girl, she had no words to tell and felt that she had no permission to talk about the assault.

She began to cry and thanked me for listening and "for teaching my children."

Her husband came into the room at this point looking for her. When he saw her in tears, he put his hand on the back of her head and began stroking her hair as he gently asked what the trouble was. She instantly whirled on him and screamed, "I have told you and told you! Don't touch my hair! Why don't you listen to me?" Then she ran sobbing to the ladies room.

Her husband stood there, dumbfounded. Then he turned to me and said, "I've always loved her hair and can't resist touching it. What's wrong with that?

When I explained her story, he asked, "What do I do now?"

By this time, the other unsuspecting parents were returning and all I could say without drawing attention to this couple's agony was, "Go and talk to her."

A year later, when I was back at that school, this same couple came to me to tell me about the change in their lives: they communicated more, their intimacy now felt transcendent, and they had joined a church community that enriched their family life.

Given how well things turned out, my only regret, when I think about this couple, is that the wife had for so many years felt unable to tell her husband the story of her abuse.

Of course, not all survivors experience such an abundance of healing. They do what they can to survive. Many constantly strive their whole lives to tell their stories, to be accepted, and to heal.

There is another global community of people who are still telling their stories today and who are still searching for healing. I'm talking about people with HIV and AIDS.

In the early 1980s when AIDS and HIV, the virus that causes AIDS, were discovered, everyone became fearful. Sadly, because AIDS first appeared in gay men, homophobia contributed to the paranoia. Some people with AIDS, or who were HIV positive, were literally cast out of their families, their jobs, and their homes. Some were driven out of their communities. Many people died alone. Among the general population, there was a widespread fear of touching anything or anyone connected with the disease. Some people were even afraid to breathe the same air as someone who was HIV positive.

As time went on and the death toll mounted, the Names Project was begun in the United States. Families and friends who chose to remain with a loved one dying of AIDS were encouraged to make a quilted memory piece.

A display of these small quilts made mostly by American but also some Canadian families came to Vancouver. I went to see it and was surprised to find volunteers standing in each room with boxes of tissues. I walked from room to room admiring over 100 quilted projects – the expert and not-so-expert stitching, the ingenuity of the quilters and their creativity. Suddenly, I came upon a hanging with the colours and the graphic design of Canadian Airlines, the company my son was working for at the time. As I read the tribute to the friend and employee who had died, I saw that his name was covered. A piece of fabric had been appliquéd over top of it, to hide it. On the appliqué was stitched the word "censored." I could not believe it. The tears began to roll down my cheeks. Here was a wonderful human who could not be named because of the stigma of AIDS. Then I began to notice more covered names on other quilts and my tears flowed even more freely. I was so grateful for those volunteers and their tissues.

In 1988, these quilts and many more were put together to form a huge quilt that completely covered the Ellipse in Washington, DC, with the White House as a backdrop. (There is a marvellous video about this display called *I Bring a Quilt,* which I highly recommend.)

Thank goodness the names on the thousands of quilts that have been made since that time are not usually blocked out and I pray that some of the names on the older quilts have now been uncovered.

The stigma associated with HIV and AIDS has not vanished, however. Just talk to any woman who is HIV positive, or to any teen who has just discovered that he or she was born with the virus. Communities still abandon HIV/AIDS victims, more properly called "persons living with HIV and AIDS."

Justice, compassion, and healing for these people – and for all those who have been hurt by sexual ignorance and abuse – sometimes seems like it's a long way off. Hearing and sharing their stories is a powerful way of communicating information, building understanding, and working at healing. It is one way we can care for these people and, at the same time, open ourselves to the possibility of transformation.

* * *

Sharing stories, as I indicated above, is an important aspect of my approach to sexual health education. My hope and my belief, of course, is that through sexual health education, we can all become more sexually mature – both an important step towards and a necessary ingredient in the justice, compassion, and healing we seek.

I am immensely pleased and grateful, therefore, that I have been invited to teach in churches, synagogues, mosques, and jamatkhanas. Besides these religious communities, many secular and professional groups – including physicians, prison officials, lawyers, and teachers – in Canada, the United States, and Japan have invited me to teach about sexual health.

Over the years, I have tried to be respectful to all, to listen carefully, and to amend anything I have said that has proven unhelpful because it was disturbing or offensive. Overwhelmingly, the response to my teaching has been positive. Even so, some people have found that they prefer a different way of expressing their understanding of wholeness and of sexuality, or that they hold a different understanding altogether. As you read this book, you may discover that you are one of these people. If that happens, please know that I commend your search for understanding. If I have been in even a small way a catalyst for your own journey of discovery, then I am delighted.

CHAPTER 1

A Word or Three about Vocabulary

When I was nursing in hospitals, many of my patients were seriously ill and some died in part because they had no education about sexual health and no vocabulary with which to ask about it. They could not talk with parents, teachers, doctors, or with lovers in any meaningful way. One man died of prostate enlargement because, as he said, "I was too embarrassed to tell a doctor that my pecker wasn't working."

I became a sexual health educator in 1975 when the parents of preschoolers began to ask how to talk with their children about babies and bodies. I always began my presentations by encouraging parents and preschool teachers to use the same "proper" or scientific words for the genitals as they would for any other part of the body, such as the elbow and the knee. In response, parents would sometimes ask, "But don't you think that 'uterus' and 'scrotum' are too big for three-year-olds?"

My answer was always a pretty simple answer: "No, I don't. They already know 'tyrannosaurus rex' and 'supercalifragilistic'!" Children don't carry the same emotional and sexual baggage as adults do. If a child has never heard any other words for those parts, "uterus" and "scrotum" are as natural as "shoulder" or "toe."

Truthfully, I think "uterus" and "scrotum" are big words for *adults* who are hearing and using them for the first time. Given that most of us didn't receive much sexual health education in school or from our parents, and given the general taboo against talking about sex that many of us grew up with, it's no surprise that one of the big challenges in our quest for maturity is learning the scientific names for the sexual parts of the body, and, even more important, how to use them *comfortably*.

I have to confess that I had been teaching sexual health for ten years before I was truly comfortable using the word clitoris. Part of my discomfort had to do with pronunciation. Was it *clit*-oris, with the emphasis on the first syllable? Or was it cli-*toris*, with the emphasis on the last part of the word, like "bronto*saurus*," as I heard one person put it? Before I could say the word, I had to be comfortable that it is pronounced the first way, *clit*oris, just the way it is spelled.

The other reason I found it difficult to use the word was that I often had to say it in the context of trying to describe the female orgasm to children. In other words, before I could really say the word *clitoris* comfortably, I had to find a way of explaining *orgasm* that felt comfortable *to me*. In the end, I adopted a wiser educator's description and modified it. I said, "It's a bit like waiting for a big sneeze – 'ah, ah, ah' and finally a huge 'atchoo' – only an orgasm feels a million times better!"

I tell this story simply to make the point that awareness is easy, but integration and behaviour changes take time and practice. I jokingly tell adults to practise saying the words over and over, perhaps while they are vacuuming – they just have to hope that a friend or neighbour doesn't walk in unannounced. One woman told me that she practised the words aloud as she was driving to work, until one morning she saw the driver next to her laughing as he watched her at a red light. She was convinced that he could lip-read. At times like this, it's good to remember that it's okay to laugh at ourselves and to enjoy our sexuality.

* * *

Vocabulary is all about communication. People are more likely to talk about something if they have the words they need to express the ideas they are trying to communicate. Likewise, they are less likely to talk about something if they don't have the words they need. For example, children who have been molested are far more likely to tell their parents or other authority figure about the incident, if they have had sexual health education and know the words for the genitals. Likewise, people are far more likely to talk to their doctor about a sexual health concern, if they know the vocabulary and are confident using it, as the story at the start of the chapter illustrates.

Vocabulary is also important when it comes to communicating effectively with our partners about our sexual likes and dislikes. For example, it will be difficult for a woman to ask her partner to stimulate her clitoris so that she can reach orgasm if she's not sure what to call it. (Most of the non-scientific, childish, or coarse names for the female genitals, such as pussy, refer to the entire vulva and not to specific parts.) The same is true if she is uncomfortable talking about her genitals in the first place.

The vocabulary we use also signals to our partners (and others) our level of maturity. Children, of course, have a great time with the vocabulary of sexuality. Initially, they may enjoy bathroom humour. Poo-poo jokes abound among preschoolers and primary children. Farting and burping also provide a great source of delight for them. To some degree their behaviour seems natural and it's fairly easy to be patient with little children who are going through this stage. It's more difficult, however, to be patient with immature *adults* who are stuck at this stage – and there seems to be no shortage of these.

Of course, vocabulary is not just a matter of using the scientific names for the parts of the body and it's not just about moving beyond infantile stages of development. I believe that the scientific vocabulary helps us to respect our bodies, our sexual relationships, and our connections to each other and to creation.

There are enough crude, degrading, and offensive sexual words in every language to fill dozens of books. For example, many of the names for penis have connotations of violence and often that violence is aimed at women. Whenever I point that out to an audience, males express astonishment, and sometimes anger and defensive guilt. They say, "I never meant it like that." "I was only joking." Or "Why hasn't anyone said this before?" Locker-room terms for the penis – such as rod, tool, gun, pistol, or cock – all have connotations of violence and do not always make partners feel safe in the bedroom.

I once met a man who insisted that "Wicked Willie" was an affectionate and harmless name for his penis. The other women in the room at the time found it freeing to be able to explain their discomfort with his nickname. "Why is it wicked? Is it doing something wrong?" asked one. Another said that "Wicked Willie" made her think of sexual assaults and gang rapes in war times.

A friend told me of being given a tour of a house by a proud new owner. As they entered the master bedroom, the man said, "And this is the pounding room."

Once these men are enlightened about their vocabulary choices, they tend to join the other men in my audiences who have said, "If I had know that that word made women feel threatened and degraded, I would never have used it."

Women in my groups are often equally stunned during discussions about vocabulary. Some say, "I've always hated that word, but my partner thinks it's sexy." Most say, "I've never dared say anything about how those words offend me. I didn't want to be seen as a prig or as super-sensitive or as a man-hater."

It should also go without saying that there is no place in any relationship – but especially not in an intimate one – for name-calling. We can all condemn derogatory hurtful ·names, but I'd like to suggest that even pet names, baby names, and commonly-used affectionate names should only be used with permission. Some women have told me that they hate being called "babe" or "honey" or "the other half," but are too afraid to tell their partner. Maybe we should heed a female comedian who said to women, "If he always calls you sweetheart, it's because he can't remember your name – leave him!"

Of course, women are just as likely to call their partners "sweetheart" and "honey," and can be just as insensitive to other infantilizing or teasing nicknames.

A sexually mature person recognizes that lovers are entitled to the hurt caused by names. Sexual wholeness means that sexually loaded words have no place in anyone's vocabulary, in any situation, if offence or hurt is caused by their use.

* * *

Learning and choosing the vocabulary we use to talk about our bodies and our sexuality goes hand-in-hand with knowing our bodies and understanding how our sexuality changes and develops over our lifetime. And so it is to these topics that we turn next.

CHAPTER 2

Adult Bodies

When it comes to our bodies, it's tempting, as adults, to sometimes take the attitude of teens who think they know it all. After all, we've lived with our bodies our whole lives. Yet whenever adults sit in on the "body science" presentations I do for children, inevitably more than a few will come forward and thank me because they learned something about their body they had never known before. We are never too old to learn more about our bodies, and it seems that there is always something new to learn.

THE MALE BODY

The Penis

It will come as no surprise that most adult males harbour some anxiety about the size of their penis and wonder if they "measure up."

This interest in penis size has given rise to many myths, such as you can tell the size of a man's penis by the size of his nose, or by his shoe size, or his body size. Let me repeat. *These are myths.*

Thirty years ago, men asked me about the penis "enlargers" that used to be advertised in the back of some magazines. Today, pop-up ads for penis enlargement patches and herbal pills – not to mention pharmaceutical aids for erectile dysfunction – litter our computer screens. These ads go to great lengths (no pun intended) to exploit men's fears while making outlandish claims for the benefits of the advertised products. A bigger penis, the ads say, will produce psychological benefits (less depression and greater self-confidence), physical benefits (stronger, longer lasting erections; greater ejaculatory volume; etc.) and romantic benefits (the ads claim that most women prefer larger penises). The message men receive from all of this is that "size really does matter." No wonder they're anxious.

Let me dispel these concerns.

First, women who have been educated about sexual health and who are sexually mature themselves know that penis size is unimportant to sexual satisfaction. Clitoral stimulation, which most women require in order to have an orgasm, is not connected to vaginal penetration, but to external touch.

I like to address the nervousness many men feel around satisfying a partner by reminding them of the saying, "It's not the size of the wand, but the magic that's in it that matters." For most women, penis size isn't nearly as important as the person to whom the penis is attached. Rather than spend your money on surgery or penis enhancers, you can be a better lover by learning about foreplay and by talking with your partner about what is pleasurable and erotic for you both.

Second, there is much less difference in penis sizes than most men think. In its relaxed state, penises come in many different sizes and shapes. Erect penises, on the other hand, are all nearly the same size. Erection is the great equalizer. So relax.

In terms of its biological function, the penis is designed to deliver sperm. Sperm are mighty swimmers, so penis size does not affect fertility. Any male can deliver sperm, even with a micro-penis. In other words, whatever length you get after you're five years old is decoration! And, if you can ejaculate semen, then personal satisfaction is virtually guaranteed.

Circumcision

Men sometimes mention circumcision as a concern. Again, my message here would be "relax." Cleanliness is the most important factor for intact foreskins. Pull the foreskin back in the shower and gently remove any smegma – the white cheesy secretions that form under the foreskin (and between the folds of the vulva) – you may find. You do not have to use soap, which can be very irritating.

Very occasionally in young males, the foreskin may become stuck in the retracted state during intense arousal. Again, relax, stand in a warm shower or bath, and gently coax the foreskin back into position as your erection subsides. Occasionally, a young male may experience some bleeding with a first-time, intense erection. Not to worry. This is within the range of normal. However, if you are worried, visit a doctor.

Some people are concerned that circumcised males do not experience as intense or as satisfying orgasms as uncircumcised males. I think that the jury is still out on that issue. However, it may be one of the reasons why many parents do not have their newborn sons circumcised, as was usual 40 years ago. If circumcision is important to you for religious reasons, become educated and be informed before making any decision.

The Testicles and Sperm

The scrotum is the bag or sac of skin that encloses the testicles or "balls." It is normal for one testicle to be bigger

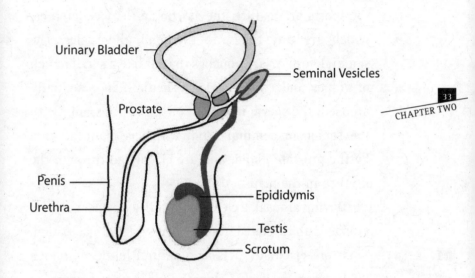

Male Reproductive System

than the other one, and for one to hang lower in the scrotal sac. I like to tell people that if God had hung them side by side, they'd bash each other to death when you walked.

Testicles make sperm, but do not store them. Once the sperm are mature, they swim up the vas deferens, which are tiny tubes, to the seminal vesicles. The seminal vesicles are pouches that sit like a small bunch of grapes under the bladder. When a man is sexually aroused, the sperm move out of the vesicles, mix with the semen or seminal fluid, which is manufactured by the prostate gland, and are ejaculated through the urethra in the penis.

During arousal, a clear liquid called Cowper's fluid is produced and secreted from the penis prior to ejaculation. This "pre-ejaculate" acts as a natural lubricant, which aids intercourse itself. Cowper's fluid may have sperm in it, which is why we call couples who use "pulling out" or "withdrawal" for contraception "parents"!

The Prostate Gland

The prostate gland is a small doughnut-shaped organ that sits at the base of the bladder. The urethra runs through the middle of it. The prostate gland makes semen, which keeps the sperm nourished.

As a rule, the prostate doesn't cause problems, but it can become inflamed by a sexually-transmitted infection. If that happens, you might feel discomfort when urinating or ejaculating, and a trip to the doctor is in order. The doctor will order a urine test (urinalysis) and do a rectal exam, which means he or she will insert one finger, suitably gloved and lubricated, into the rectum to feel for any inflammation or irregularities. This only takes a minute and you should not feel embarrassed about having it done. Doctors do it every day. So please, do not delay a visit to the doctor if you think you may have a problem. A simple visit and examination can save your life! You may not know that you have an enlargement or an infection, so some doctors do the examination on all men as a matter of routine.

As men age, some non-cancerous enlargement of the prostate is common. Men begin to feel the need to urinate during the night or to urinate more frequently during the day. Doctors can often relieve this need to urinate frequently with a relatively simple surgical procedure.

Many doctors do regular PSA testing on older men, to check for cancer in the prostate gland. The PSA (prostate-specific antigen) blood test can detect early prostate cancer. Although like many tests it is not 100 percent accurate, it can save your life, so please, be mature and look after yourself. Your doctor can also advise you about other tests that may be useful. Take advantage of modern medical care. Your loved ones will be proud of you, and thankful.

Prostate Cancer and Sexual Functioning
One of my older male friends and his wife recently told me their prostate cancer story. They both went to consult the urologist when my friend was diagnosed with prostate cancer. The urologist discussed all of the treatment options with them and the surgeon promised to do his best to maintain my friend's sexual function. Together with the doctors, my friend and his wife chose a complete (radical) removal of the prostate gland. Fortunately, all went well and if anything, my friend now says that his orgasms are a little more intense.

There are many discouraging stories out there, but remember, everyone is different so everyone's outcome is different. Just because something happens to someone else doesn't mean it will happen to you. Many people have very positive results, just as my friend did.

Self-examinations

Today we have an escalating incidence of testicular cancer in young men, aged 14 to 34. I begin to teach self-examination of the testicles in Grade 5 classrooms, because this age group is not shocked or squeamish. For these students, self-examination of the testicles is just one more health-related topic and it makes sense to "go there." As an adult, you may feel somewhat uneasy about examining yourself if you've never heard about it or done it before. But let me assure you, it's easy to learn, it won't hurt, and it could save your life.

Testicles should feel soft and rubbery, like a peeled, boiled egg, only not that big! Down one side of each testicle you will encounter something that feels like a thick piece of string. This is the vas deferens, the tube that the sperm move through to get to the seminal vesicles, where the sperm are stored.

Examine your testicles once a month. The perfect time to do this is when you are taking a shower. A testicular lump may be quite small, sometimes no bigger than a grain of salt, and it may not be painful. If you find one, go to the doctor to have it checked out. Nine times out of ten it will not be cancer, but only the doctor and an ultrasound examination can say for certain. Your life is in your hands!

Of course, if you're married or have a partner, your wife or lover can also help out by examining your testicles for you! In fact, doctors tell us that it is most often lovers who find breast and testicular lumps.

Finding is one thing. Telling our partners about what we've found is something else. It requires sexual maturity. When I taught in university classes, adults often confessed to being too embarrassed or not confident enough to tell a partner about an unusual lump or mole. This is why it's so important that we educate ourselves as adults about our bodies. The more we know about our bodies, the more comfortable we will be talking about them. And the more comfortable we are talking about our bodies, the more able we will be to care for ourselves and our loved ones. It may happen that we can save a life just by speaking up.

Are Gay Men Different?

I teach sexual health in Japan on a regular basis. From the outset, I was told that there is a strong taboo against homosexuality in Japanese culture. Yet I actually found that most Japanese were simply waiting for permission to talk about homosexuality, as well as about transgendered and intersexed people.

When I indicated that I was willing to talk, the questions came quickly. One question people asked many times was, "How is a gay man's body different than the body of a heterosexual man?"

The simple answer is that there is absolutely no physical difference between the bodies of heterosexual men and gay men. For some reason, many Japanese thought that if there was no difference on the outside, there must be a different arrangement of the internal organs.

If people are raised in a culture of suppression around these topics, it shouldn't surprise us that they will begin to indulge in this kind of magical thinking as a way of explaining things to themselves. Unfortunately, this kind of ignorance, based on a simple lack of education, often leads to prejudice and intolerance, and, in the some cases, can even lead to violence.

In 1994, Dr. Geoffrey Hopkins, professor emeritus of the Department of Psychiatry at the University of Alberta, said the following in a letter to the editor of *The Globe and Mail*:

> With reference to the outbreak of homophobia
> in the House of Commons (and elsewhere), it

is worth remembering that homosexuality is an organically determined pattern of behaviour. It is, therefore, not a perversion or disease and not amenable to treatment. It is heartening to realize, on the other hand, that homophobia is probably treatable.

Toronto lawyer Clayton Ruby wrote the following in a similar letter.

I note that the RCMP has taken the position that it will not knowingly hire gay Canadians because "most policemen are uncomfortable working with them." A similar feeling led to the persecution of Chinese in British Columbia not so long ago, and Jews and Catholics until quite recently in many occupations. It is evil.

Gay men face the same health issues as heterosexual men. They need to take exactly the same care of themselves as do others. No doctor can tell if someone is gay or straight by examining them. Don't let a lack of education prejudice your attitudes, your moral responses, or your health. Be like my Japanese students. Ask questions, become informed, and learn to celebrate diversity.

THE FEMALE BODY

In the 1970s, the Boston Women's Health Book Collective published *Our Bodies, Ourselves*. For the first time, women had a reference book that not only gave them accurate information about themselves, but made the information approachable and easy to read. There were lots of clear illustrations and the writing and reporting were done by the women in the co-op, not by doctors or other high-powered medical experts. The book has been updated and revised several times over the four decades since its first publication. I recommend it highly.

The Collective has also published *Our Bodies, Ourselves: Menopause, The New Ourselves: Growing Older*, and *Sacrificing Ourselves for Love: Why Women Sacrifice Health and Self Esteem...And How to Stop*. They are worth seeking out.

Despite the fact that accurate information has been available to women for years, there are two mistaken notions about the female sexual anatomy that I hear repeated constantly. These misunderstandings persist,

I think, because centuries of shame about our bodies have discouraged us from looking at our own genitals, let alone talking about them.

Gershen Kaufman and Lev Raphael wrote a book called *Coming Out of Shame* in which they said, "Shame is the most disturbing emotion we ever experience directly about ourselves, for in the moment of shame we feel deeply divided from ourselves." Of course, they weren't just talking about sexual shame, but that statement clearly expresses the harm done when we are denied permission to learn about and care for our own bodies.

The first misunderstanding arises because we often say, "Men (or boys) have a penis and women (or girls) have a vagina." This statement leads many people to think that girls and women urinate out of their vaginas. An amazing number of women have told me that they've been removing their tampon before urinating to protect it from urine. Some have even delayed urination for hours because they didn't have another tampon to insert.

The belief that women urinate from the vagina leads some people to believe that sex is dirty. After all, if urine is dirty, then the vagina must be dirty.

And if the vagina is dirty, then sex, which requires penetration of the vagina, must also be dirty. For millennia, women have also been taught – mostly by male religious authorities – that their menstrual flow makes them "unclean." Again, if menstruation is "unclean" and if it comes from the vagina, how can sex be anything but "dirty"?

Let's set the record straight. Males have two openings between their legs: the anus for feces or stool, and the urethra in the penis for urine and for sperm and semen.

Females have three openings between their legs: the anus for stool and the urethra for urine, which is a sterile fluid when excreted. Between the urethra and the anus, females have a vagina, which is the birth canal. The vagina is about the length of your middle finger and stretchy enough to allow for the birth of a baby. It makes moisture to ensure cleanliness, just as your mouth does. Some days, the moisture dries to a whitish or yellowish colour on your underwear. This is a sign of good health. Menstrual flow is also sterile when it drips out of the uterus. The vagina can become infected by sexual contact with a partner who has an infection, but, normally, the vagina is a clean and healthy part of our body.

The second misunderstanding also arises from the popular tendency to say, "Men (boys) have a penis and women (girls) have a vagina." Children and some adults then believe that the word vagina refers to all of the female genitalia.

When I retired from full-time teaching, my colleagues very generously threw a party and took me to see *The Vagina Monologues*. The play was a revelation that made us all quite sad. Most of the female characters were not talking about their vaginas at all. They were talking about their vulvas. We knew that the author, Eve Ensler, meant to educate as well as to entertain, but I felt devastated by the laughter of the audience in the face of such a lack of education. There was no remedy after the play but chocolate desserts and the encouragement of each other as sexual health educators.

Let me repeat: the vagina is the birth canal. You cannot see the vagina except with a doctor's speculum.

"Vulva" is the better term to use when we want to refer to the female genitalia in general. We should be saying, "Men (boys) have a penis, women (girls) have a vulva" to be more accurate and helpful.

The folds of skin that comprise the vulva and that cover the clitoris, the urethra, and the vagina, are called labia. The larger folds on the outside, nearest the thigh, are called the labia majora; the thinner ones, in the middle, are called the labia minora. They can be different colours and different sizes and be perfectly normal. Each woman is unique. Together, the labia are called the vulva.

The clitoris sits at top of the vulva, where the labia come together. The clitoris contains lots of nerve endings, even more than the tip of the penis, so it is very sensitive to touch stimulation. The visible part of the clitoris is as big as the tip of your baby finger and, like a penis, becomes erect during sexual excitement.

Of course, unlike men, women have most of their reproductive organs inside.

The Ovaries, Uterus, and Menstruation
The ovaries are the female equivalent of the testicles. Unlike the testicles, however, which make new sperm all the time, the ovaries contain, from the moment a girl is born, all the ova (the tiny "egg" cells) she will ever have. Women have two ovaries, one on either side of the uterus, which are connected to the uterus by

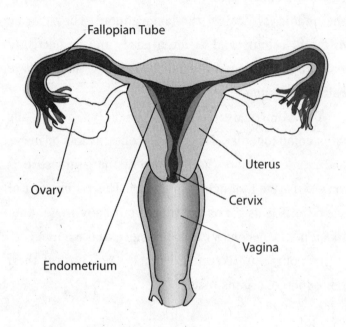

Fallopian Tube

Ovary

Endometrium

Uterus

Cervix

Vagina

Female Reproductive System

the fallopian tubes (similar in some ways to the vas deferens in men, in that they are the path from one reproductive organ to another).

Approximately every 28 days, one ovary releases one ovum. The unfertilized ovum does not come out with the menstrual flow. It begins to dissolve about 12 hours after it comes out of the ovary. It is pure protein and the body simply reabsorbs it. In fact, the ovum may never enter the fallopian tubes.

Fertilization of the ovum, when it happens, usually takes place in the fallopian tubes. The fertilized ovum then travels to the uterus, where it will attach itself to the uterine wall and begin to develop. About one-quarter to one-half of all fertilized eggs do not attach, and dissolve in the uterus.

A common misunderstanding, usually from the very old-fashioned films many of us saw when we were in school, is that menstruation is connected to ovulation, and ovulation to menses. Most females miss ovulating two or more months each year. They still have their periods, but that isn't proof that they have ovulated. And sometimes females are ovulating, but not menstruating.

The Breasts

If men are anxious about penis size, women and girls are typically anxious about breast size. Again, here are some scientific facts that may help alleviate your fears.

Breasts are designed for feeding babies and size does not matter. Once breast feeding is established after the baby is born, all breasts make the right amount of milk.

Unfortunately, in our sexually immature world, breasts are used to get men excited and to sell everything from chain saws to toothpaste, not to mention the swimsuit editions of sports magazines. When women are faced with the loss of a breast or breast tissue due to cancer, this irrational sexualization of breasts in our culture increases their anxieties about being "a real woman," or about their sexual partner's ongoing interest. Sadly, if the sexual partner is not mature, the relationship may in fact end, furthering the survivor's sense of themselves as an undesirable person.

There are days when I want to shout at our society, "Grow up! Life itself is what is important, not body parts!" Of course, losing any body part due to injury or disease bring us face to face with our mortality, and that can be a very frightening thing. But as the wise ones say, "It's what's inside that counts."

Examinations

Just like men, women need to adopt a mature attitude when it comes to the physical examinations we should all do or have done in order to ensure that we remain healthy.

Because most of a woman's sexual organs are on the inside, this means regular visits to the doctor. A pelvic exam is necessary to check your ovaries and the uterus. A pap smear (samples of cells taken from the cervix, the opening to the uterus) is necessary to test for cervical cancer.

First, however, as with males, the doctor should take a medical history. Are you healthy? Do you have any general health problems? How often do you have sex? Do you have sex with one, or more than one partner? What kind of sex do you have, and what kind of protection do you use? What protection does your partner use? Is your sexual experience satisfactory? Do you have an orgasm? And finally, do you have any pain or worries at the moment? As in examinations for males, the doctor should not assume that you are heterosexual or exclusively lesbian. Be prepared for the question and be prepared to be honest.

You should be examined with each new sexual partner, just as males should. If you are certain that your relationship is mutually monogamous, you should still be examined annually. A pelvic exam and a pap smear only take few minutes, and they could save your life.

Some women delay their medical examinations because they dislike being examined by a male physician. If this is the case for you, change doctors. There are lots of good female physicians out there. Again, be mature and take responsibility for your own health care.

This means, by the way, that you shouldn't hesitate to ask questions, to ask for explanations, and to ask for a nurse, a friend, or your partner to be present with you during the examination. You are entitled to choices and to a full understanding of why certain questions may be asked of you, and why specific procedures must be done. We all need to be sexually mature in the doctor's office because the doctor may *not* be! Take charge – it's your money and your life.

Breast self-exams

Your doctor will check your breasts for lumps as part of your annual physical, but this doesn't let you off the hook from doing your own breast self-examinations. Women should exam their breasts monthly. After a shower is a great time. If don't remember how, your doctor can give you a pamphlet that will explain the procedure. And remember, if you have a partner, you can always ask him or her to help!

* * *

Our bodies are a wonderful gift, so it only makes sense to get to know them as well as possible, and to take good care of them.

CHAPTER 3

Midlife Matters

Do you remember when you were in elementary school and you thought that anyone over 20 was old? I doubt if you still think that way today. Today, most people at midlife don't even want to think of themselves as *aging* let alone as *old*.

Obviously, our perceptions of age and of aging change as we age. Part of this may be due to the fact that life expectancies have increased tremendously in most parts of the world and the former "old" is now "midlife." But the bigger truth is that many people simply don't like the idea of getting older. For these people and this kind of subtle "ageism," I have one piece of advice. Get over it! You may not like it, but aging is normal, and although it can be challenging at times, it has lots of benefits too.

My husband has a sweatshirt that says, "A little grey hair is a small price to pay for this much wisdom." When you consider how much money people spend on hair dyes alone, not to mention on cosmetic surgery, you have to ask, "Where is wisdom?"

As we age, many of us gain a lot of satisfaction from being able to say "Been there, done that." Even more satisfying, however, is being able to say, "I no longer *want* to go there or to do that." I suspect that most of us would not want to go back even one day in our lives intellectually, or in experience, or in emotional intelligence. Yet we have great difficulty accepting that our bodies age, and that this is perfectly normal.

Although education does not necessarily lead to wisdom in this regard, it is a great place to start. Becoming educated and informed about midlife can be a great way to grow more comfortable with our bodies and with the ways they change as we grow older.

MENOPAUSE AND ANDROPAUSE

Both men and women begin to produce less testosterone and estrogen – the "male" and "female" hormones respectively – as they age. A similar decline happens with the production of other hormones, too, and much research is now being done on how all of this affects our bodies.

We call this natural aging process in women *menopause*, and in men *andropause*. I am going to write about menopause and andropause together, because there are so many similarities between the experiences of men and women at this stage of life.

Hot flashes, night sweats, avoidance of sex, and irritability are all stereotypical symptoms of menopause. Less well-known is the fact that men in midlife may also experience all or some of these same symptoms. Sadly, the symptoms of andropause are not broadly publicized and men, thinking that only women have these symptoms, often remain silent about their own experiences. One elderly man told me that he suffered through several years of hot flashes, sleep disturbances, and a lowered sex drive, all the while worrying that he was turning into a woman. Few men are mature enough or well-educated enough to talk about the symptoms of andropause they may be experiencing.

The changes men and women experience in hormone levels affect more than just sleep and libido, of course. Many women experience vaginal dryness, for example. Vaginal dryness can be relieved with lubricants and there are many different kinds of creams and gels to choose from. Try several. Find out which products feel good for you and your partner. You can have a lot of fun buying them and experimenting. Even good old-fashioned KY jelly now comes in a form that not only lubricates the genitals, but heats them as well. Are you mature enough to enter a love shop or your local drug store and search through the products?

Midlife for men sometimes means a somewhat softer erection. It may also mean that it takes longer and more direct stimulation to produce an erection, and then to ejaculate. If you are concerned, or if your problem seems more severe than this, it is always worthwhile to have a checkup with your family doctor to make certain that you are not suffering from other physical impediments.

A world of caution is worthwhile here. The "little blue pill" or its equivalent may seem to be an easy solution to a more flaccid erection, but if one's health is compromised by the drug, or if you do not address the stress that often contributes to erectile dysfunction, the sex is not going to be worth the potential damage to your overall well-being.

Likewise, Viagra and similar drugs will, by themselves, not improve a couple's sex life. There are many reasons why love-making may become unsatisfactory or problematic for one or both partners, and pills will not do anything to make these problems better without honest communication. For example, frequency of intercourse is often cited by couples as an issue that causes tension in their relationship. Introducing a drug such as Viagra may remedy the situation if it is the woman who has wanted more sex, while the man has felt unable to respond due to erectile dysfunction. On the other hand, if it is the man who has always wanted more sex, introducing a drug such as Viagra may actually aggravate the situation if having a firmer erection makes him press for sex even more. Some people have told me that they gave up using the pills because one of the partners was not interested in daily or even weekly sex. Fortunately, because they were able to talk to each other, they discovered they could to go back to cuddling and to other intimacies that they could both enjoy. As always, communication is the heart of good sex.

Marriages can go cold and infidelity can occur because one partner (or both) is not willing to recognize the midlife issues at play, or to put the necessary work into alleviating the issues, or to talking about them with their partner.

How mature are you? Are you seeking sexual wholeness? It won't happen with multiple partners or with cessation of sexual activity. True, some couples *do* stop having sex as they age, and that can be a legitimate decision for them, if it is mutually communicated and agreed upon. But I think that most aging couples *want* to have wholeness in their sex lives throughout their entire lives.

The key is communication, making time to talk, being open, and sharing with and listening to each other.

DREAMS AND FANTASIES

Besides changes in sexual desire and sexual satisfaction, both men and women have talked to me about increased sexual fantasies. One woman told me how troubled she was because she was having dreams about having sex with her nephew. She said, "I'm disgusted with myself. He's an awkward, pimply, grunting teenager. I would never dream of having sex with him in my waking hours."

I told her that these kinds of dreams and fantasies seem to be a normal part of aging for many people and she burst into tears of relief.

Judging from the evidence, many midlife men fantasize about hopping on a motorcycle and roaring off into the sunset with a young blonde riding pillion. Sadly, when a man turns this fantasy into a reality, his wife and children get left behind – and not just physically, but often financially and emotionally as well, with devastating effects that impact both his ex-wife's ability to support their children, and his children's performance in school and in other areas of their life.

We are wise, of course, not to take our night dreams literally, and we need to be cautious when deciding whether to try to live out our waking fantasies, sexual or otherwise. Most sexual dreams and fantasies are just that – dreams and fantasies. They don't do any harm and may even provide a helpful outlet, as long as we don't take them too seriously, or try to make them a reality when someone other than our partner is involved. Knowing this is part of sexual maturity.

Again, I believe that if adults were educated about midlife issues so that they could prepare themselves emotionally and intellectually for the changes midlife involves, families would experience far fewer problems and much less trauma.

STRESS

Many of the dreams and fantasies that occupy and distract men and women at midlife are fuelled by stress.

For healthy middle-aged men and women, the stress of work at this time in their lives can reach very high levels, especially if they have to travel for business.

As well, because many adults delayed their childbearing, they now find that their children are going through puberty at the same time as they themselves are dealing with their own hormonal changes. As a result, some days the whole family winds up swinging from the chandeliers.

Then there's the fact that many people at midlife find themselves taking care of their aging parents on top of everything else. Sandwiched between their parents' needs and the needs of their own children, where and how do they find the time and energy to care of themselves?

No wonder when it comes to sex many individuals and couples at midlife find it difficult to relax into foreplay and love-making.

Unfortunately, all of this stress is often magnified by irritability caused, in part, by dropping hormone levels. Both men and women complain that their partners are tired and cranky. If you ask them, children (usually teenagers) will tell you that they are constantly being "attacked" by parents who seem to have no patience for or understanding of their behaviour, and who criticize everything from their clothes, the hours they keep, and their friends, to their music and their sleeping and eating habits.

Much of this critical behaviour reflects the parents' own insecurities about their aging, disappointments in their own life, and anxieties about the future. It can also be triggered or intensified by sleep deprivation, long working hours, and lack of any meaningful communication with a partner, or with the children themselves.

Men appear to be more vulnerable than women to the extremes of this kind of behaviour. As Jed Diamond says in his book *Male Menopause*, "Men can feel cut off at the knees." Midlife crises can generate horrendous frustrations, which some fathers express through violent actions directed at themselves and at those around them. If rages, debilitating depression, or violence is happening in the home, everyone – but particularly the next generation – gets traumatized.

Again, communication is the key to dealing with these problems. Acknowledging the stressors at play and finding ways to lessen the loads can involve the whole family. Can the kids do more? Are there resources in the community to help with aging parents and disabilities? And is this the time for some counselling or therapy?

Don't forget the fun things that can help you reflect on your experience, laugh more, and gain a more positive perspective. How about a holiday, or simple things like going to a movie, attending a night of jazz, taking tango lessons, or going skiing? Is money in short supply? Gather the kids and camp in the living room for one night, tell ghost stories, and laugh at corny jokes. Or how about a bike ride, or a picnic at the beach, or even in the snow? Fresh air and exercise are cheap and tremendously restorative.

Another suggestion for taking yourself "out of yourself" is to volunteer for something you believe in or want to know more about. It doesn't have to be a long-term commitment. And you don't have to be highly skilled. Soup kitchens are glad for an hour or two of people's time. Can you peel vegetables, mop a floor? Volunteers often say, "I get more out of volunteering than I give." Volunteering can, in fact, give you a whole new perspective *and* improve your love life.

Researchers, the medical profession, community services, and public educators obviously still have a lot of work to do in this area. Faith groups could also work harder at reaching to out people at midlife. Several studies have shown the positive health benefits of attending religious services or organized events on a regular basis. Both physical and mental health can improve when people join and belong to a group.

CONTINUING EDUCATION

Clearly, there is much more to say about midlife than I can possible say in this small book. Fortunately, opportunities for continuing education in the form of classes on these issues continue to grow.

No doubt many more people will turn to the Internet for information. My only caution in this regard is to make certain that information sources you rely on are endorsed by medical and scientific organizations!

Personally, I must confess to being "old school" when it comes to educating myself. Books are my passion.

When it comes to andropause, there are two books that I can highly recommend. *Midlife Man: A Not-So-Threatening Guide to Health and Sex for Man at His Peak*, by Dr. Art Hister, is fabulous, entertaining, and educational. Women will enjoy the book too, especially the cover with the photograph of a naked midlife man. And no, it's not a photo of the author. Dr. Hister has a marvellous, quirky sense of humour and he does a superb job of dispelling myths and inspiring men and women to celebrate aging.

Jed Diamond, whom I quoted above, is a physiotherapist and well-known author. His superb book called *Male Menopause* gives extensive information in a very readable and approachable style. My favourite chapters explore the surprising parallels between males and females in midlife.

There has been a whole rainforest (renewable, we hope) of paper used to publish books on perimenopausal, menopausal, and post-menopausal women. Please visit you local bookstore and library, have a look at them all, and choose one or two with which to educate yourself. One that I love to recommend is called *Facing Changes, Finding Freedom: Canadian Women at Midlife*, by Rosemary Neering and Marilyn McCrimmon. It is an unusual book in that the first chapter is entitled "Money," surely a subject that can be crucial to healthy aging.

MIDLIFE: A SPIRITUALITY OF SEXUALITY

Midlife is often the time when mature adults begin to think about the big-picture questions about human life. This question or searching is typically spiritual in the broadest sense and can take many different forms, from involvement in a religious community to less traditional forms of religious practice.

And it's not just those who identify themselves as being "religious" or "spiritual" who find themselves asking fundamental questions about life. I must admit I was shocked recently, in a class I was taking at Vancouver School of Theology that was being taught by Douglas Todd, an internationally known and multi-award winning writer on religions. Doug said that agnostics and even atheists could be spiritual! It had never occurred to me that atheists could be spiritual. Shock and horror!

I began to read Doug's book *Brave Souls: Writers and Artists Wrestle with God, Love, Death, and the Things That Matter* and especially his chapter "The Atheists." I was struck by how many of those he interviewed did indeed express a sense of spirituality or what I would call a longing or search for spirituality. In Todd's book three well-known Canadians were quoted.

Author Mordecai Richler said, "In a sense, all my work is about a search for values or a code of honour that one can live by."

Renowned Haida artist Bill Reid said, "This world is much greater than anything man can imagine. There is no need to plaster religious illusion over it."

And author Jane Rule said, "I think what I believe is that people have to invest meaning in life."

Of course, all religions wrestle with the definitions of spirituality and what it means to live with spirituality. Leiden Museum in Zurich has a statue of the Hindu god, Shiva Nata Raja, a dancing Shiva, holding in his arms many symbols of the abundance of spiritual life. One foot is lifted high and the other is balanced on the back of a small man, crouching over a leaf. Joseph Campbell is said to have interpreted this as man, so intent on the material world that he doesn't know that a living god is dancing on his back.

All of this is my attempt to introduce the idea that our spirituality, however we define it, will influence our sexuality. As Mordecai Richler and Jane Rule say, we need values, a code of honour, and meaning in our lives, and I would say, in our sexuality as well. Bill Reid and the Hindus would say, creation is much greater than we can ever imagine so stay awake, keep searching.

Whenever we look at sexuality and spirituality together, the word morals is going to pop up.

The *Oxford Dictionary* defines morals as being "concerned with right and wrong conduct or duty to one's neighbour." It goes on to include "virtue, conscience, courage to do the right thing unmoved by odium or ridicule."

Some people would naturally ask whose ideas of right and wrong should prevail in a community, whose conscience, whose idea of the "right thing"?

Most of us, I think, would agree that honesty, responsibility, privacy, respect, safety, mutual consideration, and generosity of spirit are all aspects of morality that we would wish for ourselves and in our relationships. Some would see their spirituality reflected in those values and others may not, but when it comes to our most intimate relationships we can agree that these morals are important. All relationships need morals to survive and flourish.

So what does sexuality mean to us? The *Canadian Oxford Dictionary* says that there are three parts to sexuality: possession of sexual powers and capacity for sexual feelings, sexual desires and feelings collectively, and sexual orientation.

These definitions might lead us to ask further questions about what our families, faith groups, and cultures say about the spirituality of sexuality.

Faithful people, clergy, and institutions have sometimes held – and continue to hold – extremely negative views of sexuality. Writers who have interpreted the Torah, the Koran, and the Bible have been — and can still be — sexist, judgmental, and denigrating about sexuality.

In Douglas Todd's book *Brave Souls*, atheist Robert Munsch says, "I grew up a good, repressed Catholic — the word, the flesh, and the devil. It really mucked up my sex life. I had a bad body image. It took me a long time to realise I didn't have to be a saint — I could just be a human being. It's good to be a human being."

This kind of sexual repression has a long history in the Christian church. The early church fathers believed that sex was for procreation only and seemed to go out of their way to discourage parishioners from pursuing sexual relations at all. At one time, in fact, repression was so strict that sexual intercourse was forbidden on Sundays, Wednesdays, and Fridays. It was also forbidden for the 40 days of Lent, for 40 days before Christmas, and for three days before taking Communion. That left very few days in the year in which sex could be enjoyed, free of guilt and shame. No wonder everyone went to a glorious celebration mass at midnight on Christmas Eve – you could go home, feast, drink, and have sex!

When sexuality is understood to be sinful and shameful, then no one is allowed to talk about it, teach about it, or even think about it.

Historically, this conspiracy of silence has been deafening and life threatening, as ignorance of sexuality led to prejudices that crippled women's lives and sometimes proved deadly to their children. It wasn't until 1827, for example, that the ovum was discovered, and only in 1875 was the sperm's role in fertilization understood. Prior to that, in the 17th and 18th centuries, "spermists" believed that the sperm cells they looked at through microscopes contained the entire future person, in miniature. In other words, the woman's only part in reproduction was her uterus, which provided a safe place for the sperm to mature. It was also believed that if her she gave birth to a girl, it was because her uterus would not accept her husband's male sperm. At the time, this was sufficient grounds for a man get rid of his wife and many men did just that, including Henry VIII. At certain times in history and in some cultures, it was also common practice to kill unwanted female babies.

Today, we believe that modern medicine and the clergy of all faiths are better informed. But are they? Are we? Judgmental attitudes, embarrassment, shame, and guilt can still be used to silence and paralyze us. At the 16th International AIDS Conference in Toronto in 2006, Dr. Julio Montaner and his fellow scientists from UBC proposed that if every person known to be HIV positive was provided with anti-retroviral drugs, the disease could be wiped out in 45 years. Opposition to this common sense approach appeared to centre around costs, but, if we truly believed in a spiritual approach to sexuality, one that recognizes the value of all life, we would do it. At the same time as we hear voices of political and fiscal opposition, we also hear a litany of prejudices from some very loud "religious" voices: "AIDS is God's punishment of sinful people – drugs users, sex-workers, homosexuals, and the heathen in other countries."

If we acknowledge that the spirituality of sex touches on everything in creation, that the sanctity of life is a worthy goal, then we have a lot of questions to ask about the wider world in which we live. If we tackled all of these questions, this book would be thousands of pages long.

There are many authors – much more qualified than I am – who have written about a host of universal topics from a global, spiritual perspective that includes sexuality. Sallie McFague, a professor of theology and a prolific writer, is one I admire. Her book *Super,*

Natural Christians: How We Should Love Nature, shows the connection between a spirited sexuality and the environment, to cite one example.

Carter Heyward, writing in the newsletter of the Society of St. Junia the Apostle said this:

> The process of realizing oneself and all creation in relation to the Creator, people began to call "spirituality." The process of realizing oneself in relationship to other human beings, people began to call "sexuality."

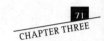
If we want to celebrate the wholeness of sex, we will take these definitions seriously, and then take a hard look at many other areas of human life that are in need of healing.

CHAPTER 4

Celebrating Our Bodies

My presentations to children and their parents always contained many positive messages about the body. Inevitably, after a session on growth and the normal changes that take place at puberty, adults would approach me and say, "Where were you when I needed you?" Often, they would go on to speak of the shame and guilt, of the hatred and distrust of their bodies they experienced due to a lack of education about what is "normal," and to having received few if any messages that affirmed the goodness of their bodies.

Girls and women especially need to hear these body-positive messages. Studies report that most women hate at least one part of their body. Is it any surprise, then, that trips to the plastic surgeon have become common for women, and even for young girls in their teens. (Lest you think from this comment that men are immune to this negative body consciousness, let me assure you they're not. Men visit plastic surgeons as well, but in smaller, though growing, numbers.)

Even more worrying to me is that fact that both women and men have told me about procrastination around visits to the doctor, for fear that the doctor would notice, comment on, or be judgmental about, a perceived physical deficit or lack of "beauty." One woman told me she had delayed her vaginal exam and pap smear, which could have alerted her to invasive cancer, because she had no time for a pedicure!

Strangely, in a world where people starve to death every day in impoverished countries, in this country we have anorexia and bulimia, conditions that can cause life-long problems, even death.

At the opposite end of the eating and weight spectrum, there is growing alarm in our society about obesity. I don't want to downplay this problem, because we *do* need to promote healthier food production and better eating habits together with exercise, for adults and children alike. No arguments there. But too many messages about health and weight blame the victim, destroy self-esteem, and produce poor body images.

I believe that if we could find a way to heal social isolation and teach better coping and social skills, we could reverse this trend toward self-defeating and self-destructive behaviour.

If only we could celebrate our bodies with joyous caressing, from birth to death. The Dalai Lama has said that the force that brings the deepest satisfaction to the world is the tender embrace between mother and newborn child.

In her thanksgiving poem "Paean," Jill Dawson celebrates her baby son's penis.

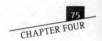

Paean

to my child

with his tiny

pod of a penis

O, how I love to

smother it in kisses,

douse it with vanilla talc:

that butter-pale catkin

of downy-soft skin.

His clear yellow urine

– I'm not taking the piss –

only meaning to praise:

smallness

friendliness.

O, at last, to love
not to envy it
– which has deflowered no one,
penetrated nothing, caused
no more offence than
a chipolata sausage. Uncooked.

To think,
all were button mushrooms once
every last one
sweet and temperate.
Such monuments I would make to it!
The Buds of Stonehenge,
Cleopatra's thimble
the Eiffel Thumb.

O, but how my son
will curse me, at twenty
reading this.
So proud will he be
of his grown up
penis.

People I have shared this poem with have said that they think Jill Dawson is very "brave" to have written it. Brave because in Western society we don't often acknowledge the sensual nature that is implicit in our love for our children.

Perhaps if we could recognize the sensuality of that adoration and be cognizant about how it differs from erotic love, then we could be more mature in our adult lives and with our adult lovers.

Some artists and writers have been able to celebrate their lovers' bodies, but most of us, I think, find it difficult. Do you have a way to express adoration of your lover's body in adult terms? What would express maturity and wholeness for you?

AGING BODIES AND BEAUTY

The common fear of our aging bodies has been especially beneficial for the cosmetics industry, for plastic surgeons, and for advertisers. Wrinkles must be obliterated; hair dyed; body hair removed; baldness cured; and drooping parts lifted, suctioned, and Botox-ed.

When I was a child, I loved my grandmother's papery skin and her white hair. There were not a lot of grandparents around when I was at school and those of us who had one or two were very proud of them. Today, perhaps because so many aging people have such little respect for their own aging bodies, young people's fear of aging is almost an obsession. It is widely believed that old age means loss of beauty and vitality.

The Bible contains an interesting story that, for me, speaks to this issue of beauty and aging. The story, which appears in Genesis 12:10–20, is about Abraham and Sarah, who were in their 70s when a famine struck the country where they lived. Abraham decided they should go to Egypt, where their prospects might be better. Before they set out, he said to Sarah, "You are so beautiful that men might kill me to have you, so let's pretend that you are my sister, so they will not kill me." The Bible story goes on to say that, indeed, Sarah was seen by the Egyptians to be so beautiful that the pharaoh took her to his palace and made her his wife for a time!

Although we might question Abraham's judgment in trying to pass off his wife as his sister, and although having to become the wife of the pharaoh was perhaps not something that pleased Sarah very much – one can only imagine the conversation they had when it was all over! – I like the story because the whole narrative turns on the beauty of this older woman. And there was no plastic surgery or Botox in those days!

Another story, this time from my teaching experiences, involves a blessing that was conferred upon my aging body by a three-year-old. I was sitting on the floor of a preschool with a crowd of little ones. Just before we were to begin, I put my hand up to still the voices. Before I could say a word, the cherub seated next to me reached up and patted the loosening flesh of my upper arm. "I love your clouds," she said. I thought it was one of the most charming and delightful things ever said to me.

A friend of mine, who been in a high-pressure job, always worried about signs of aging and spent a fortune on cosmetics and surgery. Then she was diagnosed with cancer and underwent two years of surgery and intense anti-cancer treatments. She beat the odds and today tells me that she feels blessed to have had cancer and to have survived. For one thing, she and her husband are much closer and much more intimate now, in part because she is so happy to be alive, to have wrinkles and white hair. She has even freed herself of makeup. Her husband says that, in the past, her cosmetics and hair spray made him afraid to "mess her up." This couple has learned an important lesson about aging gracefully!

AGING BODIES AND SEX

Perhaps because younger people have such difficulty seeing the beauty in aging bodies, they have even more trouble recognizing the sexuality and need for sexual intimacy of aging and aged people.

Looking at my grey hair, children would often ask me, "Do old people have sex?" I would answer enthusiastically, "Yes, many people enjoy sex their whole lives!" The common response from youngsters, and surprisingly from the parents too, was "yuck!"

Children easily understand the biological need for sex in reproduction, but because so many adults carry around the baggage of centuries of shame about sexuality, not many children ever hear about the positive aspects of an active sex life.

Parents often say that they are afraid to tell their children that sex can be fun and restorative because they're afraid it will encourage their children into precocious sexual experimentation. In fact, the opposite is true. Countless studies done worldwide show that knowledge gives self-confidence, and the ability to recognize exploitation, abuse, and unsafe sexual activity. I believe parents need to celebrate without shame adult sex lives that are safe, nourishing, and supportive. I also believe we need to celebrate the sexuality of older people, however they choose to express it.

Aging people do not have to have sexual intercourse to enjoy intimacy. Sometimes a man will suffer from erectile dysfunction due to surgery, medications, high blood pressure, diabetes, or other chronic conditions.

Medical and pharmaceutical aid is valuable if the man is mature enough to be honest with his doctors. But a number of aging and aged couples have told me that although the male partner is unable to have an erection or to sustain an erection for sex, they nevertheless have very active sex lives using many different expressions of intimacy.

Touch is one of the most important requirements for human relationships. Even when a partner is disabled with severe restrictions on physical movement, hugs, handholding, gentle massage, or just lying together can be a profound expression of love. More intimate acts of oral sex, mutual masturbation, in fact, any act of intimacy that you both enjoy is to be celebrated. Surprising to many people is the joy of simply talking with each other and the erotic responses that open-hearted sharing can create.

Perhaps a shared sense of humour is the most intimate joy. I remember my shock when I watched an explicit video at an education conference many years ago. The elderly volunteer, heterosexual couple had agreed to allow the documentary film producers to video them attempting to make love in several different places in their house. As they tried the kitchen floor, the bathtub, and finally, their bed, they used several tubes of lubricant and chocolate syrup. It was clear that their physical limitations hampered some of the positions they tried, and sometimes you could hear groans and painful gasps. But what I remember most was their laughter during filming. The smiles, chuckles, squeals of delight and sometimes tears of laughter never stopped. It was, at the time, a scandalous film, but also a non-stop celebration of physical intimacy and joy. Their bodies were no longer beautiful in a youthful sense, but their delight in each other was inspiring.

Sarah Hampson, a columnist for *The Globe and Mail*, wrote a marvellous piece in the December 6, 2007, edition exploring how midlife women feel about men and lovers of the same age. "He should feel like an old pair of sweatpants, comfortable to be around and reliable," said one 57-year-old woman. Several women commented on how status in business or society no longer interested them. The ability to be mature (even about an ex-wife) was far more important than sexual love-making or intercourse. Ms. Hampson quoted from a book entitled *Senior Prom: How Survivors of Long Marriages Can Successfully Find New Partners*, by Pat Hutchens. According to Hutchens, "even impotence is taken in stride. There's far more to intimacy than coital sex."

Another woman in Ms. Hampson's column reported being sad when a long love affair ended, "not because sex was hot, but because the loving, the tenderness was amazing." Hampson ended the column by saying, "They understand that at this age, the naked body is not a show of vanity... The act of undressing with someone else is a beautiful display of vulnerability."

Of course, some elders will mutually choose not to be sexually active. That is their choice. But for those who choose to continue to practice the "sacred communion," please continue!

One aspect of elder care that has always bothered me happens when care facilities separate partners of many years. A couple may have been together for

50 years and yet they may placed in separate beds, separate rooms, even separate facilities. Are caregivers so inhibited, so immature, that they cannot risk seeing a couple in bed together?

One of Canada's earliest feminists in the public arena was June Callwood, a journalist and activist who was passionate about many worthy causes. I saw an interview George Stroumboulopoulos conducted with her, on CBC's *The Hour*, just a few short weeks before she died, in 2007. Both George and June acknowledged that she was near death. They both seemed at ease and June responded seriously, honestly, and sometimes with humour to his many questions about her life, her family, and her work.

Near the end of the interview, George asked June if her relationship and the intimacy in her marriage had changed now that she and her husband knew she was dying. She began her reply by suggesting that a long marriage has about seven marriages within it. I'm going to re-create her comments as best I can from memory.

She said, "There is the honeymoon marriage at the beginning." Then she laughed and said, "Well, that doesn't last very long!" She went on to talk about the marriage when the babies are coming; then another, different kind of marriage as the children are growing up. Another kind of marriage occurs once the children are grown and perhaps both partners are out in the community building their career and are very busy. Then comes the retirement marriage and the grandparenting marriage. Finally, comes the end-of-life marriage. Intimacy is defined differently at this stage. There's much more deep sharing, and talking takes on a new intimacy. Cuddling and handholding become much more intimate. And then June laughed heartily and told George that her husband had said to her, just a day or two before, "You can't die yet, you still have a nice bum." What a superb example of sexual wholeness continuing throughout a life-long relationship.

ROMANCE

Falling in love can happen at any time and even at age 95 the brain will release oxytocin, a hormone that will make you feel like a teenager again. There is tremendous variability in individual people about what is deemed to be attractive in a partner, and these preferences can change over time. As people age, they find physical characteristics to be less important.

They look for kindness; openness; listening skills; and the ability to give, share, and receive with grace. Our sexual drive has always been in our heads, not in our genitals, and some take longer than others to recognize that.

The Internet is becoming popular among seniors as a place or way to meet other seniors to talk with about sexuality, or for flirting, for dating, and yes, for finding a new partner. The Net is anonymous, accessible, and the possibilities for meeting one's needs are boundless. The opinions expressed by seniors online vary from "Sexual intercourse is not at all important to me," to "I want someone with round heels." The Net is also a good meeting place for aging people who are any orientation but heterosexual.

Of course, when it comes to the Internet, the usual caveats apply for seniors as they do for all ages. Be aware that there are fraudsters, deviants, and exploiters online who see seniors as easy targets. Take care and go slowly into a serious relationship. And, if in doubt, run!

One other risk in elderly relationships that surprises younger generations is that of heartbreak if the relationship ends. The elderly can suffer just as much as any teenager can and will need support to survive the tremendous disappointment that ending a relationship can bring.

SEX DURING ILLNESS AND DISABILITY

Our sense of our sexuality and our sexual relationships can be sorely tested when we are ill or injured.

I remember hearing Dr. George Szasz, a doctor who specialized in spinal cord injuries, say that the most common, first question asked in the ER by young men brought in from motorcycle crashes was, "Am I ever going to have sex again?" He said that, at first, he was embarrassed by the question and used to ignore it.

Several years later, however, he noticed that nurses were charting the question, because it kept being asked. So he forced himself to answer, "Yes, we are going to do everything we can." And a strange thing happened. He began to observe that those men who received an affirming answer made a faster and more determined recovery than other men who were ignored, or who were too shy to ask the question in the first place. Once he realized this, he began to train doctors and nurses to answer the question. Then he went even further and developed a new medical specialty, focusing on sexuality and the disabled. His pioneering work enhanced and saved many lives.

Clearly, our physical well-being, our sense of self, and our sexuality are intimately tied up with each other. Almost always, our first response to illness or disability will be to perceive them as a threat to our sense of self, and that in turn threatens our sexuality. Or maybe, as with the men who were in motorcycle crashes, it's the other way around. Illness and disability threaten our sexuality, and this in turn threatens our sense of self and our ability to recover.

But it doesn't have to be this way.

My friend Francis is shining example of someone whose sense of self and sexuality remained undaunted by illness. During the bald days of her chemotherapy, I met her at a local shopping mall. She was bubbling over and almost dancing, she was so full of the joy and anticipation of entering her new favourite store, Tie Rack, to buy another scarf for her new scarf collection. As we talked, she laughed all the way through stories of shocking friends and neighbours as she tried new styles of swathing her head and herself in scarves. It was as if her friends were thinking, "How can you be so sexy, so sensual when you're bald and fighting for your life?" Her husband, Ken, is a man of quiet chuckles and I can see him, sitting back, laughing with her and saying, "You go, girl!"

We can also *choose* to do things to our bodies that *might* be perceived as threat to our sexuality, but which aren't necessarily so. I remember how proud my family was of my niece Miriam, who had a lifetime growth of long, dark beautiful hair shaved off to make a wig for a child with leukemia. Perhaps because her sense of self has been so strongly nourished, her sexuality was not compromised by weeks of baldness. What's more, she was able to educate many of her friends and the people she works with about "wigs for kids with cancer" – all with the support of her boyfriend, Toby.

MODESTY, PORNOGRAPHY, AND NUDITY

In Paul Loeb's book *The Impossible Will Take a Little While*, Victoria Stafford tells a story about the Pine Ridge girls' basketball team, quoting from Ian Frazier's book *On the Rez*. The girls faced an obviously hostile and racist crowd before a game in Lead, South Dakota. Fourteen-year-old SuAnne led her team out onto the gym floor. Then, all alone, she performed the Lakota shawl dance and song in Lakota – "graceful and modest and show-offy all at the same time." The crowd became silent, their hostility silenced, and at the end they applauded.

I have not seen the Lakota shawl dance, but somehow I doubt that it is anything like the dance of the seven veils. Erotic dances may have a place in a private bedroom, but what I love about the Stafford story is the word *modest*.

Modesty is rarely celebrated these days and I believe that immodesty, especially in clothing, has become a negative force in the Western world today.

London's Victoria and Albert Museum opened their new Jameel Gallery of Islamic Art in 2006. The gallery houses many spectacular works of art that reflect the Muslim belief in order, goodness, and unity in creation. One work in particular speaks to me of how modesty can enhance sexuality. The piece in question is a ceramic tile, which depicts some beautifully but modestly dressed picnickers in Iran. They are all fully clothed, but that only adds to their mystery and allure.

Schools and workplaces alike struggle with dress codes and seem to be singularly reluctant to use words such as *modesty* and *dignity*, let alone words and concepts such as "respect for one's school, job, or firm."

And do scantily clothed models really increase the sales of everything from cars to deodorant?

Of course, no one wants to go back to Victorian times, when pianos were covered with shawls to hide their legs, but I believe that modesty in clothes for males and females could do a great deal to aid our search for mature and healthy sexual relationships.

The Internet has opened another arena of extreme immodesty. Couples may mutually agree to film each other in erotic poses or activities and that may be fine, as far as it goes. But I believe the pictures become pornographic when a breakup of the relationship occurs and one of the disgruntled partners posts these images or films on the Internet. What makes these images pornographic, to my mind, is that they are no longer private, but are publicly displayed without permission.

Pornography is especially problematic for women it seems. Women who have talked to me about their partner's addiction to pornography tell me that they have two problems. One problem concerns their feelings of physical revulsion: "Why is my body not enough for him? Why is he always looking at other women?" Their self-esteem is shattered. Then they tell me that they fear for the relationship itself, especially if the man will not acknowledge his addiction or talk about it with her. And, of course, the hours that he spends looking at pornography is time taken away from the family, the care and maintenance of the home, the garden, the vehicles, and the everyday chores. Friends of mine who are therapists tell me that addiction to pornography is now the number one reason couples seek marriage therapy.

Pamela Paul has written a book that should be required reading for every adult. It is entitled *Pornified: How Pornography Is Transforming Our Lives, Our Relationships, and Our Families.* I recommend it highly.

A number of people have pointed out that pornography is sometimes made by and for women. Andrea Dworkin, in her book *Heartbreak*, says, "It is not equality for women to use porn the same way men do. The world gets meaner as prostitution and pornography are legitimized. Now women are the slave population, an old slavery with a new technology, camera and camcorders."

Is there something to be said for nudity? Yes, indeed. Just as I am suggesting a return to higher standards of modesty and dignity, I would suggest that there is or should be room in our society for nudity.

We in North America are finally maturing about children and nudity in the summertime. The wisdom of preschoolers who strip off wet bathing suits amazes me. Who wants to spend hours in wet clothes? It seems we still have some distance to go, however, before we will allow nude bathing beaches for adults. It is time we grow up and stop becoming hysterical over appropriately designated nude-bathing and tanning.

The English-speaking world has had difficulty accepting nudity in art from time to time. Recently, a thought-provoking statue of an older naked man with suitcases was erected in a public area in Penticton, British Columbia. It was almost immediately vandalized. Assuming that a stereotypical conservative elderly person would not be out in the dead of night attacking sculptures, I think it's safe to assume that at least some younger people are uncomfortable with nudity too. And whom do we blame for this: their parents, their schools, their faith groups, for failing to help them see the beauty in naked bodies?

It is said that beauty is in the eye of the beholder. That aphorism recognizes that we all have different interpretations of what we see. *Cahoots*, a women's magazine published in Saskatchewan, used a painting of a nude woman on one of its covers. The artist, Kal Barteski, painted the woman in varying shades of red. The response from women was astonishing – everything from adoration to hatred, from reasoned analysis to disgusted gut reactions. The editors were very surprised by the strength of the women's voices, both pro and con, and they were wise enough to print them. Real truth includes all truths.

If we could develop a wholeness about sexuality that honoured the human body in all its forms, then we could critique art and perhaps come to some consensus about what is art, what is erotic, and what is pornographic.

From my perspective, erotic art is designed to provoke a sexual response but is done with the models' or volunteers' or actors' full consent and no one is exploited. It involves adults only and is produced for a targeted audience who can give informed consent to view it.

Pornography is exploitive and/or abusive – it compartmentalizes body parts and the participants are forced to be involved, either by threats of violence or through more subtle means, such as drugs and alcohol, or even money. Questions of legality and organized crime often arise. The number of deaths in the pornography industry is rarely publicized. Participants struggle with addictions and with the related health problems; with STDs, including AIDS; with feelings of shame and disgrace; and tragically, with suicide.

TOUCHING BODIES

During World War II, countless babies and children were abandoned or orphaned. After the war, the

institutions that were supposed to care for them were overwhelmed. Doctors began to notice that babies who were rarely touched, except for the most basic of care, failed to thrive and some even died. As more studies of touch were done in the years that followed, researchers observed that lack of touch was a problem, a life-threat for all of us. The elderly in care facilities; patients, especially children in hospitals with severely restricted visiting regulations; the disabled and the mentally ill all showed failures to thrive, diminished immune systems, chronic and severe infections, and premature death.

We all need touch and when we get it some remarkable things can happen. I remember, for example, seeing a television program that described the discovery of researchers that even unnoticed touch increases positive feelings and – surprise, surprise – honesty.

When a coin was left in a public telephone, the person who found the coin always gave it back to the researcher who rushed up to the finder and touched the person's arm while asking, "Did you find my dime?" If the researcher did not, ever so lightly, touch the finder's arms, the coin was *not* returned. In fact, the finder even denied having pocketed the dime.

In another experiment done at a university library, some of the librarians were asked to subtly touch a borrower's hand as they returned their books. The rest of the librarians were told to avoid any touch at all. When the researchers questioned the students about the library staff – "Were they helpful, attentive, friendly?" – the students who had skin contact all replied in the affirmative. The untouched borrowers gave either neutral or negative replies.

We are all different in our need for human touch. My family of origin was of the Anglo "stiff upper lip" school. My siblings and I were rarely hugged beyond babyhood and we are not huggers even now! But the hugs I have received from friends during a crisis have sustained and strengthened me. I have never forgotten them.

One afternoon, after tea with one of my very closest and oldest friends, Jony, the phone rang as were saying goodbye. Jony stood there, in my kitchen, listening to me and realized that it was the hospital calling to say that my son had been hit by a car. She immediately wrapped her arms around me and held me upright as my knees buckled. I was so very grateful not to be a heap on the floor. She not only preserved my dignity (very important for my stiff upper lip!), but those few seconds of physical support enabled me to carry on. My son made a good recovery and I still remember that hug.

So many people say, "I don't know what to say, so I didn't go to the hospital...," or "I didn't visit her at home... I didn't go to his funeral... I avoided meeting her at work..." But the truth is, when people are going through a time of crisis or struggle, you really don't have to say anything. Often, a pat on the hand, a rub of the shoulder, even the smallest touch can heal.

I find it so sad that our raised awareness of child abuse and sexual harassment has stopped us from touching each other, especially since there are lots of ways to touch that cannot be misconstrued – placing arms only on the shoulders, pats on the back, the holding of a small hand on the way to the nurse's room. Other safeguards can be put in place for teachers, such as windows on the inside walls of classrooms. Of course, before giving one, you should always, always ask, "Do you need a hug?"

This latter instruction is a safeguard for adults, too, even same-sex colleagues or acquaintances. Ask, and if the answer is "no," accept with good grace. We are not all the same. You can always ask if there is anything else you can do. And remember, just the asking can be comforting. Bodies are sacred and everyone names what is sacrosanct for them.

CHAPTER 5

What's Normal?

Maybe there was a time in human history when everyone agreed that heterosexuality was normal, that sex in bed in the missionary position was normal, and that anything else was abnormal. Well, maybe there was such a time and maybe there wasn't.

I believe that one sign of maturity, sexual or otherwise, is the ability to accept ambiguity and diversity. I also believe that most people who demand security and "normal" behaviour in others do so out of fear. They lack a sense of security themselves, perhaps because of abuse, trauma, or repression, or maybe because they lack experience in the broader world or education about diversity.

One of my favourite questions is, "Who gets to say what is normal?" – especially when it comes to sex. Some people say that oral sex is not normal, yet many studies reveal that 93 percent of North Americans have tried it and about 80 percent enjoy it on a regular basis, including, I'm told, the majority of gay men. Studies also suggest that a minority of gay men – and more heterosexuals! – enjoy anal sex. Many couples have sex standing up or in countless other positions. Who says what's abnormal?

HOMOSEXUALITY, BISEXUALITY, ASEXUALITY

Homosexual, heterosexual, and bisexual orientations appear to be congenital – an orientation one is born with, not a choice one makes later in life. Yet homosexuals and bisexuals have typically been ostracized, or worse, been persecuted by our society. Given that non-heterosexual orientations have had such a bad rap, is it any wonder that many gays, lesbians, and bisexuals suppress or deny their orientation throughout their lives, or only "come out" later in life?

There are now several international research studies going on to learn more about asexuality. One of these studies is being conducted by Anthony Bogaert, a psychologist at Ontario's Brock University. Bogaert wants to know if asexuality is an authentic orientation on a par with heterosexuality, homosexuality, and bisexuality, or is it a disorder? He estimates that there are 3.5 million asexual people in North America now.

Asexuality means never feeling sexual desire for another person. One woman described her lifelong absence of sexual urges as "liberating," in a Can-West News Service story entitled "Asexuality on the rise as lust loses its lustre," which appeared in the *Vancouver Sun* in April 2006.

Although able to develop crushes, based on emotional interest, she says sexual desire – toward either gender – never enters the picture.

"I think it's in my hardwiring because it feels as normal as being right-handed or blue-eyed," she says.

"I didn't really think about it until suddenly everybody [in my youth] started speaking this whole new language. I thought that eventually I would think just like them. But I'm 43 now...."

The official Nonlibidoism Society, fronted by a young woman in the Netherlands, similarly explains that asexuality "doesn't mean that 'you don't like sex'; a nonlibidoist has not had a sex drive ever."

Although asexual people do not engage in sex, they might teach the rest of us quite a bit about intimacy.

It is possible that asexual people may enjoy being in a mature, committed relationship as much as sexually orientated people do. Asexual people may enjoy the same intimate styles of touching, caressing, and other expressions of love involving touch, on which everyone thrives. Just because they have no sexual desire does not mean that they are without the emotional or physical need for touch.

My plea would be that we accept asexuality as an honest and perhaps congenital condition no different than any other orientation. It would be unfair to push asexual people to marry and to have children (perhaps to give us grandchildren), or to patronize them saying, "It's a phase, you'll grow out of it," or "You'll change your mind when you really fall in love."

CELIBACY, SINGLES, AND SEX

Celibacy is a choice that some singles will make. The word originally referred to the unmarried state, which may or may not have included abstinence from sexual activity. In modern times it usually means abstinence *and* unmarried.

Celibacy may be a very deliberate choice for religious reasons. Nuns, priests, and monks of many religions are asked to take vows of celibacy. People may also choose to be celibate if they experience no desire to be sexually intimate, as in the case of someone who is asexual.

Some people, of course, don't have sex because there are no sexual partners available to them. These people are not celibate per se. Celibacy implies a deliberate choice to *abstain* from sex, even when it's available. Rather, it's better to speak of these people as being sexually inactive.

Celibates and people who are sexually inactive due to circumstance are not without sexuality. Both may suppress desire or sublimate it into other activities, but they still need to care for their bodies and for their sexual health.

In our culture, perhaps because of the prominence of sex and sexuality in the media, we tend to assume that the vast majority of people want to have sex, and the more often the better. Yet even among sexually active single and married people, sex isn't necessarily a top priority. In an amusing but seriously done piece of research, 38 percent of Canadian women surveyed said they preferred chocolate to sex, and 20 percent of the men surveyed agreed that chocolate was better than sex! French sexologists have reported that 47.5 percent of people living alone couldn't care less if they went without sex for months on end, and 23 percent said they would be relieved.

The same could perhaps be said about marriage. We tend to assume that the vast majority of people *want* to get married. Yet in Japan, men are reporting *Renai Ken-o Sho* (dislike of love relationships) and the number of loving couples in the country has plummeted. In an August 6, 2006, article entitled, "Facing Middle Age with No Degree, and No Wife," *The New York Times* reported that an amazing number of men between 35 and 44 years of age are single and not unhappy! The men who were interviewed gave a variety of reasons. Some said that they'd never met "the right one"; others said they did not feel financially secure enough to enter into a marriage relationship. The article went on to say that they all looked younger than their ages and all reported satisfaction with their lives.

Clearly, we need to include celibacy and singleness in our definition of what falls within the realm of normal sexual and relationship choices.

CHILDREN

But what about children?

One of the challenges sometimes put to celibates, singles, and asexuals is that they are denying the "natural" or "normal" desire to have children.

But is it really "normal" to want to have children? Most cultures certainly pressure people to reproduce. Even so, perhaps because it's a little easier to speak up and say who we are these days, more and more heterosexual couples are declaring that they don't want children. That being the case, maybe we should say that there are many kinds of normal. It may be normal to want to have children, but let's also say that it is normal not to want children.

I don't believe that there is a divine plan or an innate biological urge that drives everyone to reproduce or to be sexually active. I believe the idea that we all want to have sex and that we all have biological clocks and are driven to have children is cultural.

In our culture, we sexualize children from the time they are born. Well-meaning adults coo over little children, saying to the parents, "All the girls will be after him," or "Keep your shotgun oiled, Dad." Barbers tease boys about girlfriends; girls' magazines headline articles on how to attract boys.

When they're in their 20s and 30s, young adults are pestered with questions about marriage and children. I know couples who suffer agonies protecting their privacy about infertility or about their desire to remain childless.

I have a radical idea for you to consider. Our sexual responses are not always oriented toward our genitals and our reproductive organs. I believe that God or Allah or Yahweh calls us to live in communities, to care for each other, to work together, and to participate in the raising of children. But not everyone has to or is meant to reproduce!

Isabel Carter Hayward is one of my favourite theologians. She wrote a grace poem about bread. In the poem, she speaks of planting the wheat, nurturing the plants, harvesting, milling, and finally, making the dough and baking. This poem symbolizes, for me, our call to community, that we all may eat and have equal power to be who we are, and not be forced to be who others think we should be.

MASTURBATION

Is masturbation normal?

Masturbation is a normal, healthy choice for those who desire a safe sexual outlet. The old belief that touching your genitals will make you blind, bald, and insane has been dispelled, even for those of us who wear glasses, lose our hair, and are considered slightly wacky (usually by our children)!

To be sure, the belief that masturbation is a sin, a grave moral evil, is still around in some quarters. Fortunately, there are many other voices of reason and balance we can choose to listen to. Dr. John Theis, of St. Jerome's College, is one of those. In a 1986 article for SIECUS (Sexuality Information and Education Council for the United States), he wrote the following.

> We have come to know over the years that sex is not bad and that there is nothing inherently evil about masturbation. We have also come to the awareness that there is no value in coercion, and so, if masturbation is not appropriate for a given person that is their prerogative.

All that I can say is "amen."

Masturbation can be a means to release tension, to learn more about oneself, and of course it brings pleasure. Researchers have noted that women can experience more intense orgasms with masturbation than with sexual intercourse. Both men and women appreciate the pleasure masturbation can bring at those times when they feel they might otherwise have to push their partner for intercourse. God gave us bodies to enjoy in many different ways. Masturbation is one way to affirm our sexual needs.

SEX TOYS

Just as there is nothing wrong with masturbation (as long as you are not staying home from work in order to masturbate!) there is nothing wrong with sex toys either.

And that goes for adults of *all* ages! A woman in her 80s approached me after a public presentation on sexuality one day and shyly asked if I knew where she could buy a vibrator. She explained that her husband of more than 50 years had died and she was now living in a seniors' home. She had her own apartment, but was enjoying the company of other seniors at meals and on organized outings. She said that some of the other women had advised her to get a vibrator.

I told her about a shop owned and staffed by women, who would be very discreet and helpful, explaining and demonstrating the many choices. She wrote to me later saying that she had a lovely time at the shop and that she'd learned a lot. She also told me that the women friends at her seniors' home had promised each other that if one of them died, the others would remove the vibrator from the bedside table quickly, so as not to shock anyone! An excellent plan!

A word to the wise about sex toys. Please remember that they do need to be kept clean and that although many couples enjoy using sex toys, the need for cleanliness is sometimes forgotten in the afterglow following the passion.

SEXUALLY TRANSMITTED DISEASES

Sexually transmitted diseases (STDs) are not something we should ever want to call "normal," but they are common.

Because we live in an "ageist" society, we tend to think that STDs are only a problem among the young. But STDs can be a problem in the elderly, too, and are perhaps an even bigger risk for them precisely because STDs are often overlooked as a possible cause of trouble by so many doctors and families who do not expect seniors to be sexually active.

Some middle-age children rejoice when mom or dad finds a boyfriend or a girlfriend after being widowed. One woman told me that it was such a relief to have her once lonely, depressed mother in a new relationship, because her mother's spirits were high, she was taking great care with her appearance, and she was more interested in her family and in the world around her.

When I asked if both her mother and her new partner had been tested for STDs, she laughed and said, "But they were both married for more than 50 years."

Wise people know that not all "happily married" people are faithful, and STDs do not always have symptoms. Surgeries and blood products, and even transplanted organs, carry a risk of transmitting disease. It is always best to be tested and have peace of mind. Respecting each other means being mature enough to go for testing.

Recent statistics bring this point home. British Columbia statistics show that between 1997 and 2006, the incidence of gonorrhea among those over 60 has grown. In 2005, the Public Health Agency of Canada reported a rise in HIV infections amount persons aged 50 and above, from 7.5 percent between 1985 and 1988, to 13.5 percent in 2005. The agency also reported that both midlife persons and seniors suffer from serious misunderstandings and dangerous misinformation about HIV transmission, and about the effectiveness of condoms (only 13.2 percent of older women at risk insist that their partners use condoms).

Seniors living in care facilities may be particularly at risk for several reasons. If the staff or the families have no understanding of seniors' sexuality, the secrecy of sexual activity can make taking precautions problematic. The ability of seniors to give informed consent to sex is an area fraught with concern, in cases where dementia or injury maybe present, or where communication is lacking.

Seniors with homosexual orientations are also at tremendous risk, if they are hiding their orientation, or conversely, if they are being open but risking censure from the staff and other residents.

Parkwood Hospital in London, Ontario, includes over 400 beds for Canadian veterans. The staff has worked hard to develop an institutional culture that respects the needs of residents for sexual expression. This enlightened example, reported in the winter 2007 edition of *Facts of Life*, the newsletter of Options for Sexual Health, in Vancouver, British Columbia, needs to be repeated in every care facility.

CONCLUSION

Today, more than ever, we need to recognize that there is no one-size-fits-all when it comes to sexual orientation or even to the desire to have sex. There is no "right" or "wrong" choice when it comes to the question of marriage and having children, except for what is appropriate for each individual or couple.

Likewise, many of the taboos and sexual practices that used to raise eyebrows – such as masturbation or the use of sex toys – we now know are common and healthy expressions of human sexuality.

Truly, there are many ways to celebrate our sexuality. Let's be done with ignorance and judgment, so that we can all make appropriate, informed, and healthy choices.

CHAPTER 6

Marriage and Divorce

Marriage and family isn't for everyone, but it's still the choice of most adults. Even so, marriage has become the focus of much controversy and debate in recent years, particularly in relation to the question of gay and lesbian marriages.

One of the positive offshoots of this controversy is that many people have begun to learn about the history of marriage.

We tend to think of the "traditional" marriage as being one man and one woman legally joined for life. Many religiously conservative people, in particular, like to talk about traditional family values and to point to the Bible to support their claim that the "traditional" nuclear family is normative.

Yet even a casual reading of the Bible shows that the nuclear family as we understand it today simply didn't exist in biblical times. In fact, the Bible notes at least seven different types of "marriage," including polygamy (where a man has more than one wife), marriage with multiple wives plus concubines, Leverite marriage (where a man marries his brother's wife if the brother dies, regardless of whether or not the man is already married), and political marriages.

In an essay published in the *Vancouver Sun* in 2005, Professor John Klassen, from Trinity Western University in Langley, British Columbia, outlined the many changes that have occurred in marriage over the course of time. In particular, he notes the change from Greek, Roman, and even earlier times, when women were chattel – possessions or property – to be given away in marriage by their fathers. In contrast, today many brides walk "down the aisle" unaccompanied, as a sign of their free agency in marriage. Clergy may ask both the bride and groom's parents to stand and affirm their blessing of the union, but the notion of dad "giving away" his daughter is now as much about sentimentality as "something old, something new, something borrowed, something blue."

Professor Klassen also points out that the medieval requirement that the married couple have sexual intercourse in order for the marriage to be valid became a problem for the church in respect to Mary and Joseph, since Mary was supposedly a virgin at the time of her betrothal to Joseph and remained so until

Jesus was born months after they were married. To solve this problem, the couple's "I do" came to signify the completion of the contract. According to Klassen, "Sex for procreation continued to be important in the church's eyes, but no longer was it decisive in making a marriage."

The point I'm trying to make with all of this, and the point that Klassen is trying to make, is that opponents of same-sex marriage "cannot point to an enduring changeless notion of the family" or of marriage.

Torontonian Rob Steiner wrote an essay entitled "The marriage debate's at the heart of what makes a person whole," for *The Globe and Mail* in February 2005. Rob wrote the piece in response to a previous article that urged readers to distinguish between ethics and morality when it comes to same-sex marriage – ethics being a human construct, and morality, at least in the eyes of the other writer, being divine. In his response, Steiner says much of what I believe is crucial to our understanding of marriage today. Many who eschew marriage as the government's intrusion into their relationship will affirm the essence of spirituality and sexuality that Rob writes of in this piece. With Rob's permission, I quote from his article at length.

I take religion and God seriously, and I agree: Ethics and morality are different.

But I'm not sure that [anyone]...really knows more than any other human about the laws of morality that guide this universe. Morality, or goodness as the ancients called it, is just too large for any single human mind. It is a divine creation and, like God itself, it is beyond easy description.

"So I suggest," to quote Plato when he hit on this same problem 2,500 years ago, "that we forget about trying to define goodness itself for the time being."

Instead, let's seize this moment in our national life more humbly.

The reality is this: Morality is something we all spend our lives just trying to figure out. It's why we read, go to movies and worship. It's why we talk with friends and lovers late into the night. It's why none of us with young children really knows we got the answer right when they ask us, "why this?" and "why that?" It's why human beings suffer, and why we grow.

Just as scientists explore the physical laws that guide the universe, all human beings explore the moral laws that guide the universe.

But we do get hints.

In this divine game of moral Marco Polo, we do have some idea of when we're "hot" or when we're "cold." Those hints are in the quality of our relationships.

When relationships feel rusty, hard and strained, we may be heading away from morality. When we connect, deeply, with another individual, we have found some hint of the moral laws that guide the universe.

And this is why the question of marriage before us today is so profound – not just for Canada, but for humanity...

The question of same-sex marriage is all about the most profound relationships. When two human beings are able to link their souls to one another, they have found a hint of the moral laws that drive the world.

People who love so deeply that they will marry have discovered one another's truth and honoured it with their attention. They have taken the hard step of exposing their own vulnerabilities to another person and – "against, despite their will" as Greek playwright Aeschylus put it – have allowed themselves to suffer in the presence of another human being.

They have become wise through the blessing of another person's silent mouth, eager ear and yearning heart. As the Jewish mystics might have put it, the love between two human beings – whatever their gender – lights a spark in which the divine shows itself to the world.

And the hallmark of that divine communion of a married couple is precisely what those who preach "morality" lack: An ability to truly listen in the presence of another person's yearning.

I am not gay.

I am not particularly close to any gay or lesbian couples.

I don't know much about morality.

But I am a husband.

I am slowly learning – "despite, against my will" – something about love.

I have learned that the theologian Martin Buber was probably right to say that when "one responds as a whole person, one can have confidence that one can not have in any universal prescription of morality."

And I know that in the life of a human being – gay, lesbian, or straight – marriage has the power to make one whole.

As Rob Steiner says, "morality is something we all spend our lives just trying to figure out." Thomas Moore echoes that thought in a broader sense in his book *The Soul of Sex: Cultivating Life as an Act of Love.* Writer and psychologist Moore says that he approaches sex as a lover of mysteries, and that sex is infinitely more mysterious than we imagine it to be.

Let's celebrate what we do know of the wholeness of sex and marriage, and also celebrate the mystery, the life-long journey with each other as we explore them.

LUST

Is there a place for lust in all of this? Is lust part of sexual wholeness between couples?

Matthew Fox is a well-known American theologian and writer. In his book *Sins of the Spirit, Blessings of the Flesh*, he says that without lust, families would not exist. He goes on to say that lust is, in itself, holy and sacred. Our sexuality is not a problem of lust. On the contrary, our sexuality can be a path to the divine.

Fox goes on to say that sexuality can be a problem when it turns into an addiction, "but when we have developed skills of letting go and letting be and becoming emptied, sexuality does not overtake us as an obsession." This writing deserves a loud amen!

The poem called "The Lover," by Solveig Von Schoultz, seems to me to be saying similar things about lust.

The Lover
My eyes want to kiss your face.
I have no power over my eyes.
They just want to kiss your face.
I flow towards you out of my eyes,
a fine heat trembles round your shoulders,
it slowly dissolves your contours

and I am there with you, your mouth
and everywhere around you –
I have no power over my eyes.

I sit with my hands in my lap,
I shan't touch you and I'll never speak.
But my eyes kiss your face,
I rise out of myself and no-one can stop me,
I flow out and I'm invisible.
I cannot stop this unfathomable flowing,
this dazzle that knows neither end nor
  beginning –
but when at last you turn your eyes towards me,
your unaware, questioning, stranger's eyes,
I sink myself back into my hands
and take up my place again under my eyelids.

To me this poem speaks volumes about lust, sensuality, and sexuality. We probably have all had the experiencing of seeing someone "across a crowded room" that we find attractive and lust after. The question is, how do we handle that lust given our responsibilities, our obligations, our spirituality, and our search for sexual maturity.

Karen Armstrong, another well-known theologian and author, wrote in a *Guardian* essay about Yan Hui, a favourite pupil of Confucius. One day, Yan Hui told Confucius that he could not remember anything that Confucius had taught him.

"What do you mean?" Confucius asked uneasily.

"I sit quietly and forget," beamed Yan Hui.

Instead of being dismayed, Confucius acknowledged that his pupil has surpassed him. The intellect, he explained, could only "tally things up," but the deepest core of the human being, whence enlightenment comes, is vacant and receptive. "The way is found in emptiness. Emptiness is the mind's fast."

Karen Armstrong points out that the idea of deliberately starving our mind to achieve greater spiritual acuity is repugnant, even frightening for us.

I would suggest that if we could learn the value of holding ourselves in silence waiting to discern when action is appropriate and when forgetting is more appropriate, we could recognize lust for the natural emotion that it is. Then we could rejoice in our humanness, but know that our lust can be forgotten or set aside if it is not fitting.

One more reason I love his poem is that there is no lusting after good looks, rugged handsomeness, or great beauty. By comparison, I have always been uncomfortable with the *Song of Songs* in the Bible, because the lovers go on and on about their lover's beauty. Not everyone is handsome or beautiful by the standards of the day. Still, the *Song of Songs* is a glorious celebration of lust and sexuality and was a much needed reminder of the gift of sexuality in the centuries of repression.

We need to celebrate the lust that we feel for our partners, even as we recognize that lust is not an overpowering, uncontrollable force. We are not at the mercy of our hormones. Judeo, Christian, and Islamic scriptures all tell the story of David and Bathsheba. David's lust for his neighbour's wife may have been natural, but if he had been able to hold himself in silent waiting, acknowledging his human response to female beauty, he would have been able to put aside that lust as irresponsible and inappropriate.

Lust is often confused with love. How often have you heard, "I didn't mean to fall in love with my workmate, my friend's spouse, my professor..."? It is difficult for some adults to understand that lust is the first sexual response to another person, but that love takes much longer to develop and to mature.

In today's culture of trivializing sex, young people can become cynical about love, especially when they see their parents fall victim to the negative power of lust for someone else. Consider the following, written by Harold Kushner in his book *When All You Ever Wanted Isn't Enough*.

> I am afraid that we may be raising a generation of young people who will grow up afraid to love, afraid to give themselves completely to another person, because they will see how much it hurts to take the risk of loving and have it not work out. I am afraid that they will grow up looking for intimacy without risk, for pleasure without significant emotional investment.

There are many indications that Kushner's prediction has already come true. Of course, teens also have difficulty knowing what is infatuation and what is love, just like their parents.

If we could talk openly about lust and love from the time our babies are born, or before we conceive, or when we marry, or when we are growing up, we could help each other make wise choices throughout our lives. Perhaps then we would act on our spiritual or moral beliefs and not on our hormonal responses.

DIVORCE

Having said that, I need to say that not all marriages are meant to last forever.

How many times have you heard someone say, "Divorce is too easy these days – the slightest little difficulty and young people think nothing of divorcing"?

I do not agree that divorce is too easy. I have listened to hundreds of people talk about their experience of divorce in the course of my teaching and not once did I think that the marriage breakup I was hearing about was easy, or that it was a mistake or that the couple involved should have stayed together. Divorce is an awful tragedy, especially when there are children involved, but it is never an *easy* decision. It involves tremendous heartache and often affects the families of both partners.

There are many reasons why divorce happens. People change, goals differ, not everyone ages with grace and dignity, addictions become intractable, abandonment happens, or controls become freakish.

I have not ever met an adult whose parents divorced who wished they had stayed together despite constant fighting. Children generally want their parents to be happy and peaceful. If that cannot happen within the marriage, then children will typically support the divorce. They also typically want to stay connected to both parents, assuming neither was abusive. The hardest thing for a child is losing a parent through divorce.

One of the biggest challenges when a marriage ends is to recognize where the personal faults lay, to work on them, to celebrate the good parts, and to care for the children.

When a relationship fails, honesty is the most important ingredient in moving forward. For anyone who considers him- or herself to be a spiritually oriented person, being honest about the reasons for breaking up a relationship should be paramount. Lying, deceit, hiding, and denials all add terrible trauma to the separation. Couples do grow apart, grow differently, develop differing goals, and yes, sometimes meet someone else!

Divorce may be the most difficult tribulation we ever have to survive. The challenge is to survive with our moral values and with whatever sexual wholeness we have as intact as possible.

Past sexual abuse or exploitation that has not been dealt with is sometimes a contributing factor in the breakdown of relationships. Survivors of abuse are not always believed and some are even punished for reporting the abuse. This kind of response is certain to silence the survivor and tends to make them very reticent to see a therapist or a counsellor.

Shirley Tarcotte is a survivor of horrendous abuse who tells her story in an anthology edited by Brenda Lee Brown called *Bringing It Home: Women Talk about Feminism in Their Lives*. Shirley has not only managed to achieve a high level of healing despite several broken adult relationships, but counts herself blessed as a survivor. She has even moved on in her journey to the point that she now reaches out to other survivors.

Shirley demonstrates her extraordinary wisdom about the wholeness of sexuality in her writing.

I liked it when I heard that women were
capable of being strong, had a right to say

"no" and "yes" and sadly, that they too could be abusive. I wanted also to hear that not all men were bad, that they too were victims of patriarchy and violence.

I worried that good people of both genders were being torn apart and alienated from one another, and that our resources for change were being eaten up in the process. Women were being told we could have and do it all and were getting thoroughly exhausted trying. Men were being told that they were intolerable jerks and losing their confidence. I fervently believed that all of humanity was in this together, that men needed to help change the imbalance in order to live more fully, and that, for the health and growth of our children, we needed goodwill on all sides.

That quest for unity and balance belongs to us all, doesn't it? And there is hope. We have seen so many changes for the better in the last few decades.

CHAPTER 7

Sexual Maturity at Home and Abroad

I think it is far better for children and teens to know that their parents enjoy having sex than to know that they fight.

Children and teens constantly tell me that they want to learn about sexuality at home, from their parents. The parents constantly ask, "How do I talk to my children?" Or they say, "I can't possibly talk to them; you do it for me."

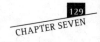

One of the common questions I get from parents of young children is, "What do I say if our children catch us having sex?" I tell parents that it is important to stay calm and if the child is very young, simply putting them back to bed is fine.

If the child is older and they ask, "What are you doing?" I advise parents not to show anger or embarrassment. Simply say, "We were having sex. That's what grown-ups who love each other do sometimes."

"Can I stay and watch?"

"No, it's private and when you're 35 and having sex for the first time, I won't ask if I can watch you." As you might imagine, a sense of humour saves the day.

Another question parents frequently ask is, "What do I say if my child asks if my husband (or wife) and I still have sex?"

Isn't it funny how we all want our children to grow up and have fine sex lives, but so many of us pretend we don't have sex ourselves?

I know that it was not politically correct, but I hugged the mother who told me of this conversation with her son.

"So, Mom, you and Dad just had sex twice, for me and Allison; right, Mom?"

Mom replied, "Yes, but you have to do a lot of practicing sex, too."

What a celebration!

Actually, you would probably be surprised to know just how many children have told me that they have crept down the stairs and watched their parents making love on the couch, or have remained unseen and unheard in their parents' bedroom while their parents have had sex. When I hear these stories, I say, "You are so lucky to have parents who love each other." This comment always results in smiles on the faces of the kids.

Mature adults are not ashamed of having sex and giving wholesome messages to children about the joys of sex can benefit them for the rest of their lives.

Ask yourself what messages you want to give your child. It might be helpful to hear what John Robinson, an English bishop, said in court about D. H. Lawrence's book *Lady Chatterley's Lover*: "What I think is clear is that...Lawrence is trying to...portray that the sex relationship is something essentially sacred...as in a real sense an act of holy communion."

TEENS AND SEX

Parents of teens often struggle with the question of how to teach their kids about sex, responsibility, values, and safety. The messages we give our young people can set the tone for a lifetime of mature responses and the wholeness we want them to have.

One story may be helpful here. A group of mothers approached me at an elementary school. They introduced themselves as neighbours, each of whom was from a different faith or culture, but all cared deeply for their families and their community. They told me that a bright and popular teenage girl, who had babysat for all the families, was now pregnant. Another neighbour was having a baby shower for this girl and all of the children she had babysat and their parents were invited. The girl was going to live at home and raise her child with her parents' help. These women wanted to honour their religious and cultural beliefs - no sex before marriage. Should they boycott the shower?

I encouraged them to put aside any judgments of the babysitter - a new baby should always be welcomed, especially since the grandparents were willing to provide a loving home. At the same time, I told them that this could be a heaven-sent, teachable moment to talk with their own children about their beliefs, their faith, about sexuality, and yes, the trials of being a teenage parent.

I suggested that they ask their children about their dreams for the future. How do they plan to get there? What will they need, and how would a baby complicate it all?

I admitted that the teenage girl may have made a mistake, but I also pointed out that condemnation and isolation would not reverse the mistake and could even be life-threatening if it forced her to leave her support system, or to make a fear and guilt-ridden decision to try to abort the child.

"Attend the party," I told them. "Enjoy the company of your neighbours and celebrate the baby. Be glad for teachable moments."

I adore the Christmas season on many levels: the music, the good cheer, the winter weather, the decorations, and oh, those glorious lights!

You'll know that I am a sexual health teacher when I tell you that I see Mary as an honourable teenage mother. I love the angel messenger and Mary's response to the news of her pregnancy. But my favourite part of the story is the Wise Men, who have come from afar, following their scientific instinct about the star. They did not expect to find a baby in a stable. Yet, without hesitation, they opened their saddlebags and gave the babe their finest gifts of gold, frankincense, and myrrh.

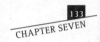

Every child, whether it is a baby or a teen, is a gift to be celebrated. The great thing about teens is that, for those who have had good teaching and who have not been exploited or have had abuse ignored, their optimism and joy about their future relationships and marriage is marvellous to behold. They are full of confidence and are not afraid to ask questions. They carry a healthy curiosity to all their activities, and their expectations for fulfillment are contagious.

This is the gift they give us, but it grows from the gift we first give them – a willingness to model and celebrate the goodness of mature sexuality in our own lives and homes.

HOME

"Home" means many things to many people around the world. Its actual structure can be of canvas, bricks, wood, steel, leather or hide, straw or mud. The furnishings may be stylish and expensive, or shabby but well-loved. There are hundreds of variations to the structures we humans call home and the best homes may cost very little.

But the word home also refers to something larger and more important than the structures we live in. Home has a deeply personal meaning for each of us. The feelings or emotions we experience when we think of home depend very much on our experience of our family life as we grew up.

Though it is, unfortunately, not true for everyone, one of the basic characteristics we often associate with home – and often sentimentalize – is safety. Most of us assume that home is a safe place, that we can trust our parents, siblings, and extended family. Yet the very presence of the ancient story of Cain and Abel in the Bible – in which Cain kills his brother Abel – tells us that, from the very earliest days of the family, the reality has not always lived up to the ideal.

Today, we constantly strive to overcome this legacy of family dysfunction to achieve the ideal of nurture, protection, and sanctuary that so many of us associate with and desire for the family.

In this regard, I am as much a seeker for the ideal as the next person. Our sexuality is such an enormous part of who we are, who we will become, and how we live our lives in the world. I believe home should balance our striving for a spirit-filled sexuality, with our base instincts. We need to recognize hurt, anger, disappointment, vengeance, and jealously for what they are – normal human responses to the breaking of relationships. But that darkness can be overcome when we learn and model appropriate coping skills, take the time to reflect on the significance (including the spiritual significance) of our actions, and learn to forgive not just our nearest and dearest but ourselves as well, and move on.

Sue Bender, in her book *Plain and Simple: A Woman's Journey to the Amish*, says that the Amish quilters love the sunshine and shadow quilt pattern because it uses dark and light fabrics to symbolize spirit, and form to create one glorious unity. The colours need each other. The balancing of opposites gives a quilt its strength and beauty.

Louise Silk wrote *The Quilting Path: A Guide to Spiritual Discovery through Fabric, Thread and Kabbalah*. She says, "Life's work is to wake up. We are obligated to know life's nature and let it teach us what it will."

Home is surely where these obligations, this waking up to both our light and our darkness, is to begin and where it is to be nurtured.

Home is where our wakefulness in regard to our sexual maturity – as well as many other things – can be challenged within a safe environment, and can be encouraged by nurturing parents and partners. We need to be wide awake, knowing both ourselves and the realities of the wider world, as reflected in the homes of others. Balance and unity may not always exist in any given moment, but it is always something we can work towards.

BROADENING OUR HORIZONS

We all benefit when our families, homes, and local communities are healthy, but we need our global community to be healthy too.

I have been teaching sexual health in Japan since 1999. Occasionally, a member of an audience will say, "There is a traditional Japanese saying 'Don't wake the sleeping child.'" They ask, "Isn't teaching about sexual health waking them to learn about sex and become sexually active?"

My message in Japan is that the children are already awake. They see the most horrid, violent pornography on TV from a very young age. They see business men reading pornographic comics on the trains. The lack of sexual maturity among adults astonishes me.

In his book *The Soul of Sex*, Thomas Moore says, "The soul of sex is not to be found only in the act of love, but also in a life motivated by a broader life and extended pleasures."

I believe this profound wisdom expressed by Moore can be applied in a multitude of areas. There are so many tragedies related to sexuality happening in the world today and we need to care about them. Africa springs immediately to my mind.

It should come as a surprise to no one that the people of the African continent are suffering one of the worst pandemics of HIV/AIDS anywhere in the world. To date, there has been a frightening lack of response from African governments, a plague of ignorance about HIV and sexual health, and unfathomable resistance to change from the churches and the conservative population.

To be fair, we must also hold up the very courageous individuals, community groups, and organizations who have tried to stem the rising tide of infection. These include, for example, Nelson Mandela and Archbishop Tutu, the many public health nurses and doctors at the local level, and the many grandmothers' groups across Africa supported by organizations such as Stephen Lewis' Grandmothers to Grandmothers.

Sometimes, though, the only way to encourage change is money. Take South Africa, for example, where studies indicate that up to one-third of the work force on any job site may be HIV positive. In a 2006 double-page report, *Globe and Mail* reporter Stephanie Nolen wrote about mining giant Anglo American, Daimler Chrysler South Africa, DeBeers, and other South African companies who have discovered that teaching their employees about HIV/AIDS has big economic paybacks.

In order to retain their workers, keep them healthy, and avoid the huge cost of constantly training replacement workers, the companies began to "broaden" their employees' lives and the life of their companies. They now offer anonymous HIV testing, counselling, and wellness programs. Not only does this education help to prevent the incidence of disease, it also helps takes away the crippling stigma attached to the disease. These companies have also begun to offer treatment that includes the anti-retroviral drugs that have not been provided by government health care in the past, and that the unemployed cannot afford.

Money talks, as the saying goes, and for those South Africans who have lost their traditional homes and now call DeBeers or Chrysler "home," economics has provided safety, sanctuary, a light in the window, and at least a warmer heart than was there before the dollar spoke.

Stephen Lewis, in a CBC sponsored Massey Lecture entitled "Race Against Time," said, "I live in hope...but I also live in rage... I cannot abide the wilful inattention of so much of the international community, the heartless indifference, the criminal neglect of people who should still be walking the open savannah of Africa."

Stephen Lewis is right to castigate so many of us for our "wilful inattention," and our clinging insanely to old rules. To cite just one example, anti-abortionists in the U.S. government refuse to give contraceptives to Third World countries for fear that the contribution would then free up money in those countries for abortions!?

As sexually mature adults, we cannot allow ourselves to sit idly by while so many people in the world suffer and die from lack of sexual health education and basic health care. It is time for us, as sexually mature adults, to awaken and to oppose sexual injustice wherever it occurs.

We are all part of one human family, after all, and we all deserve better.

CONCLUSION

Let's Celebrate!

I have tried to make this book fun, a celebration of
sexuality and of my deep belief that sexual wholeness
is available to all. How can we celebrate this gift of
wholeness?

I feel a bit like a wedding planner compiling a list
of jobs to be done, arrangements to be made, people
to contact and to contract with for the celebration. As
with any celebration, we have so many choices. Will
it be a small, quiet affair with witnesses chosen from
the lobby of city hall, or a moderate gathering of close
friends and family? Or will it be a huge gathering
with so many guests that the bride and groom are not
acquainted with them all? What resonates with you?

Of course, we can have absolutely private celebrations. Maybe we simply take the time to appreciate
fully that perfectly baked pie or hot cup of jasmine tea.
Or maybe we let ourselves fill with awe when we see
nature's miracles – the first snowflake of winter, the
first crocus of spring, a flock of geese winging over-
head – on a solo walk around our neighbourhood. But

never forget the private joys of bodies too – including the very fact that you have one!

The truth is, we can have small celebrations every day of our lives. A baby is born, a senior dies after a long and productive life, flowers bloom and leaves fall: each a chance to celebrate life, and death as a part of life, colour, and growth.

When you light the Sabbath candles, the Advent candles, birthday candles, or even a candle for your bath, celebrate your own sexuality. Those birthday candles especially remind us of what Matthew Fox said; we wouldn't be here without sacred lust!

Small, seemingly insignificant celebrations give us the confidence to take part in larger parties. Encouraging your child's school or your faith group to provide sexual health education for everyone is a form of celebration. You don't have to do the teaching yourself, but you could organize a fundraising event to pay for a professional educator, or you could make the coffee or be a greeter.

Tackling the evil of pornography, sexual slavery and exploitation is not always as risky as you might imagine. Pioneer sexual health educator Sol Gordon said, "Pornography is a symptom of society's unwillingness to promote responsible sexuality education at home and in the schools." We can so easily feel powerless when we try to face alone a huge industry that seems impervious and Teflon-coated. But imagine the celebration that you and a few others could have if you managed to remove even one piece from that wall of pornography.

Shared celebrations don't have to involve such weighty and serious matters, of course. They can also be had for the sheer fun of it. My niece Erin and I now live many miles apart, but we continue to share our joy of life and sensuality by watching each December for the first house with a Christmas tree in the window, and then we call each other with glee. Laughing with your partner about a silly quarrel or misunderstanding, sharing a goofy mix-up with a colleague at work, helping a friend through a crisis – all of these things reinforce our connectedness. When we feel accepted and cared about, our sense of sexual wholeness is strengthened mightily.

SHARED LEARNING AND HEALING

On one of my teaching trips to Japan, my hostess invited me to visit her home. Imagine my very pleasant surprise when her home turned out to be in a Buddhist temple, where she lived with her priest husband and child. At 7 p.m., we gathered in the temple to accompany her husband as he performed the evening prayers. Often, he would strike an iron bell or bowl. That sound felt incredibly sacred to me. It symbolized for me a shared and nearly silent meditation, sensual and celebratory.

Buddhist's talk about *bodhichitta*, the awakened heart of unconditional love. It is the motivation for mindful-living. As I understand *bodhichitta*, it has many dimensions, among them taking responsibility for how we express our sexuality through our actions, being committed to cultivating responsibility, and learning ways to protect the safety of individuals, couples, families, and society. In other words, *bodhichitta* always leads to healing.

So much healing that *could* be done is often left undone because we don't know how to do it. That is why I want to affirm the call to *learn,* as articulated by the seekers of *bodhichitta*. Shared learning, in my experience, is much richer and more enjoyable than learning alone. I have had the experience of distance education, where text and assignments arrive via a distant professor or tutor. Although I could do the work more quickly and race through a course more efficiently studying on my own, I missed the company of other students. That getting-to-know-one-another process that happens in a group, the telling of stories, the shared cups of coffee, the opening of hearts and spirits is a powerful and wondrous form of sharing.

Once we have learned what will bring healing, we need to take action that will lead to transformation. Another word for healing could be transformation, for no healing happens without a transformation of some sort. This, too, is part of *bodhichitta,* of "cultivating responsibility" and working to protect "the safety of individuals, couples, families, and society." There a lots of ways to do this. Write a letter, send an e-mail, start a petition to express your abhorrence of pornographic materials, sexism or racism in the media. Oppose any denigration of sexuality that comes to your attention.

Never underestimate the power of constituents' voices to a politician. There is an old aphorism that says "You can't legislate morals." What nonsense! Of course we can. Slavery was ended by legislation. Public lynching, hate speech, sexual harassment, flogging and many more have all been ended by legislation, and if they have not been entirely eliminated, at least we now consider them to be immoral. Speak up quietly or loudly, but use your power.

Nelson Mandela said, "Our greatest fear is not that we are inadequate but that we are powerful beyond belief." Don't let fear of your power to bring healing hold you back.

I would like to end this book with a traditional blessing I hope will speak to you about wholeness and sexuality.

May the blessing of God rest upon you,
May God's peace abide with you,
May God's presence illuminate your heart
Now and forevermore!

BIBLIOGRAPHY

MEN'S HEALTH

Bigelow, Jim. *The Joy of Uncircumcizing*. Aptos, CA: Hourglass Publishing, 1995.

Diamond, Jed. *Male Menopause*. Naperville, IL: Source Books, 1977.

Hister, Art. *Midlife Man: A Not-So-Threatening Guide to Health and Sex for Man at His Peak*. Vancouver: Greystone Books, 1998.

Ritter, Thomas J. *Say No to Circumcision*. Aptos, CA: Hourglass Publishing, 1992.

WOMEN'S HEALTH

Boston Women's Health Collective. *Our Bodies Ourselves: A New Edition for a New Era*. New York: Simon & Schuster, 2005.

– *Our Bodies Ourselves: Menopause*. New York: Simon & Schuster, 2006.

Cobb, Janine O'Leary. *Understanding Menopause*. Toronto: Key Porter, 1993.

Hyman, Jane Wegscheider, and Esther Rome. *Sacrificing Ourselves for Love: Why Women Sacrifice Health and Self-Esteem and How to Stop*. Freedom, CA: Crossing Press, 1996.

Neering, Rosemary, and Marilyn McCrimmon. *Facing Changes, Finding Freedom*. Vancouver: Whitecap Books, 1993.

FAMILIES

Gordon, Sol and Judith. *Raising a Child Responsibly in a Sexually Permissive World*. Holbrook, MA: Adams Media Corp., 2000.

Hickling, Meg. *The New Speaking of Sex: What Your Children Need to Know and When They Need to Know It*. Kelowna, BC: Northstone, 2005.

— *Boys, Girls and Body Science: A First Book about Facts of Life*. Vancouver: Harbour Publishing Company, 2002.

SEXUALITY AND SENIORS

Blank, Joani, ed. *Still Doing It: Women and Men Over Sixty Write about Their Sexuality*. San Francisco: Down There Press, 2000.

PORN

Paul, Pamela. *Pornified: How Pornography Is Transforming Our Lives, Our Relationships, and Our Families.* New York: Times Books, 2005.

SPIRITUALITY

McFague, Sallie. *Super, Natural Christians: How We Should Love Nature.* Minneapolis: Fortress Press, 1997.

Michaelson, Jay. *God in Your Body: Kabbalah, Mindfulness and Embodied Spiritual Practice.* Woodstock, VT: Jewish Lights Publishing, 2007.

Moore, Thomas. *The Soul of Sex: Cultivating Life as an Act of Love.* New York: Harper, 1998.

Todd, Douglas. *Brave Souls: Writers and Artists Wrestle with God, Love, Death and the Things That Matter.* Toronto: Stoddart, 1996.

MASTURBATION

Dodson, Betty. *Sex for One: The Joy of Selfloving.* New York: Crown, 1974.

GLOBAL

Adams, Vincanne, and Stacy Leigh Pigg, eds. *Sex in Development: Science, Sexuality, and Morality in Global Perspective.* Durham, NC: Duke University Press, 2005.

Brown, Terry, ed. *Other Voices, Other Worlds: The Global Church Speaks Out on Homosexuality.* London: Darton, Longman, and Todd, 2006.

GENERAL

Bender, Sue. *Plain and Simple: A Woman's Journey to the Amish.* New York: HarperCollins, 1989.

Blackburn, Simon. *Lust.* Oxford: Oxford University Press, 2004.

Dawson, Jill, ed. *The Virago Book of Wicked Verse.* London: Virago, 1992.

Loeb, Paul Rogat, ed. *The Impossible Will Take a Little While: A Citizen's Guide to Hope in a Time of Fear.* New York: Basic Books, 2004.

Other interesting and inspiring titles
from Wood Lake Publishing
www.woodlakebooks.com

The Spirituality of Nature
Jim Kalnin
ISBN 978-1-896836-87-4

**The Spirituality of
Grandparenting**
Ralph Milton with Beverley Milton
ISBN 978-1-896836-86-7

The Spirituality of Wine
Tom Harpur
ISBN 978-1-896836-63-8

The Spirituality of Bread
Donna Sinclair
ISBN 978-1-896836-85-0

The Spirituality of Pets
James Taylor
ISBN 978-1-896836-81-2

The Spirituality of Gardening
Donna Sinclair
ISBN 978-1-896836-74-4

The Spirituality of Art
Lois Huey-Heck and Jim Kalnin
ISBN 978-1-896836-78-2

The Spirituality of Mazes & Labyrinths
Gailand MacQueen
ISBN 978-1-896836-69-0

The Spirituality of Music
John Bird
ISBN 978-1-896836-88-1

All books in *The Spirituality of...* series are fully illustrated in colour with art and photos. They make fine gifts.

Next in the series, available February 2009
The Spirituality of Sex
Susan Ivany and Michael Schwartzentruber
ISBN 978-1-896836-90-9

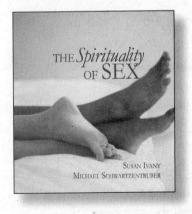

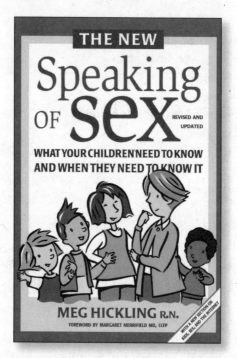